Self Test Self Treat

THE POWER TO HEAL YOURSELF

by

N.R. Gairdner, M.A., H.D.

TFT Advanced Practitioner

www.NRGHolistic.com

SELF TEST - SELF TREAT
the power to heal yourself

How to self-muscle-test accurately using the NRG Method™ of self-muscle-testing, and how to use some basic Callahan Techniques® Thought Field Therapy® protocols to successfully self-treat, resolving emotional, physical and spiritual distress, and the perturbations of life.

by

N.R.Gairdner, H.D.

© 2011

Cover image & drawings by Dana Doyle

Note for Librarians: A cataloguing record for this book is available from Library and Archives Canada at www.collectionscanada.ca/amicus/index-e.html

ISBN – 978-0-9869131-0-5

Printed in Canada
♻
on recycled paper

FIRST
CHOICE
BOOKS
www.firstchoicebooks.ca

"Norma Gairdner's method of self-muscle-testing is one of the few that have shown reliable results, and is a fine objective method of testing."

Roger J. Callahan, PhD.
Founder – Thought Field Therapy

TABLE OF CONTENTS

THE PURPOSE OF THIS MANUAL IS THREE-FOLD:

1 to explain and instruct in the correct use of the **NRG Method** of self-muscle-testing, and…

2 to show how to employ some basic **Thought Field Therapy (TFT)** protocols and algorithms, in conjunction with the **NRG Method** of self-muscle-testing, for the purpose of self-treatment with TFT, to resolve trauma, grief, phobia, and emotional distress, and a myriad of physical, emotional, and spiritual symptoms resulting from and accompanying the various stresses, traumas, toxins, and sufferings of life.

With the ability to self-muscle-test accurately, comes the ability to self-treat successfully. Although this manual employs some basic TFT protocols to assist you to self-treat with TFT, its main purpose is to teach you how to self-muscle-test. If you want to become skilled in TFT, you will need to attend formal TFT classes, many of which you can find at www.rogercallahan.com .

All TFT treatment protocols mentioned herein are used with permission, and taken from Callahan Techniques ® Thought Field Therapy ®, and based on the discoveries of Roger J. Callahan, Ph.D.

3 This manual is purposely written in such a way as to assist you to more easily learn and integrate the self-testing technique. As the story line and history regarding TFT and the NRG Method unfold, it contains specific material intended to make the instructions, which begin on **page 41**, easier to understand and follow. This is especially so if you have not studied TFT before. Although it's possible to skip the storyline and history and go straight to the self-testing and self-treating instructions, you will gain a deeper understanding and find the method easier to master if you read the entire manual once through from the beginning - after that, you can refer to specific testing and treating instruction pages, as needed.

It's good to be patient with yourself when learning this technique, and especially when self-treating. Sometimes you will need to repeat a treatment more than once (even over and over if such is the case) until you get the exact result you're seeking. There's always a way to achieve the result you want, and it's the tenacity of your intention that will lead you to success in self-treatment, and to feeling better and more like yourself than you may have felt in a very long time, or ever.

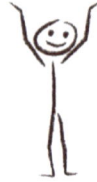

OK - get ready to go for it!

SELF-TEST SELF-TREAT
the power to heal yourself

Once upon a time there was a man who wanted to know all there was to know. He was getting on in years and was at a juncture in his life when he could do anything he wanted to do.

What he wanted to do was to know all there was to know. And so to that end, he set out on a journey to an ancient monastery in the far reaches of the world where he could immerse himself in studying and learning in peace and quiet.

He traveled for many months until he finally arrived at an old stone monastery nestled into the craggy rocks of a mountain slope.

He approached the big wooden door and knocked.

Eventually, a very old and bent-over man dressed in robes and holding a wooden staff opened the door.

"What do you want?" asked the old Master.

"I want to know everything there is to know." said the man.

"Everything....?" said the Master.

"Yes," said the man. "Everything."

The master smiled and said: "Come in..."

…well, before I go on with this story (I promise I will ☺), let me tell you about the first time I came across a reference to the brilliant and healing technique known as Thought Field Therapy. It was during an airplane ride. I was browsing through a copy of "Psychology Today" when a small ad caught my eye. The ad was for a video called the "Five Minute Phobia Cure", and although I had no phobia of my own, as a Homeopath I was certainly interested in anything that claimed to be a cure for phobias - and even if the claim turned out to be only half true, a fifty percent improvement in a phobia in only five minutes was worth looking into. I took down the phone number, and within a few days had ordered the video which would arrive in time for Christmas. Perhaps I could view it before giving it to a colleague who was studying NLP (Neuro-linguistic Programming) at the time.

I had never heard of Thought Field Therapy (TFT) and apparently had only picked up on the words "Five Minute Phobia Cure", because when the video arrived I was expecting to see some sort of new and improved version of a "phobia reframe" which I had learned back in the '70's from an old friend who lived at Esalen and who had attended Bandler and Grinder's first NLP workshop. What I saw in this little video, however, was something quite different. I was fascinated.

The moment the video ended, I called the 800 number on the back of the cover to see if I could find out more about whatever this method was, and luckily, Roger Callahan, PhD., the discoverer of Thought Field Therapy, answered the phone himself. I had no idea it was he at the time, however, and simply assumed he was a receptionist or a sales clerk.

I introduced myself as a Homeopath in Toronto, and said I had just finished watching the "Five Minute Phobia Cure", and wanted to ask a few questions about the technique.

"Fire away," he said in a jolly tone.

"Well, first of all", I asked, "Is this NLP?"

"Hell, no it's not NLP", he said, equally jolly. "It's TFT."

"I've never heard of it," I said. "Where does it come from?"

"I discovered it!" he said proudly. (*Oh my gosh, it's Dr. Callahan!*)

"Wow. Is it as effective as it looks in this video?" I asked.

4

"Hell, yes!" he said, laughing out loud.

"Will you teach me how to do it?" I asked.

"Sure I will", he said. "Come on down here!"

That was my very warm, fun and friendly introduction to TFT and to the gifted, enthusiastic and intellectually voracious Roger J. Callahan, PhD., who has since become a much respected and admired mentor, friend, and TFT colleague.

II

I decided to keep the video for myself, and told my friend he'd better get ready to learn something new and amazing.

I watched the video a few more times during Christmas week. On New Year's Eve, I went to an annual party where there was dancing and card playing and lots of healthy food and family fun.

A few minutes into a hand of cards, a neighbor friend sitting across the table from me asked what I'd been up to lately. I told her I was learning how to do a 'five minute phobia cure'.

"Well," said a very tall and hefty stranger to my left, who I later learned was a Qi Gong instructor, "Can you cure *my* phobia?"

"What sort of phobia do you have?" I asked.

"Fear of heights," he said, without looking up.

Feeling encouraged by the fact that the TFT video had used fear of heights for the demonstration of a phobia cure, I said: "Well, we can try it, if you like."

"OK" he said, folding his cards and withdrawing from the game without the slightest hesitation.

III

It was early in the evening, and no one seemed to mind the interruption, so I decided to give it a try, mostly for fun - or so I thought. As we turned our two chairs to face each other, some of the others put down their cards to watch what we were doing. At that point I think we were all thinking of it as some sort of entertaining parlor trick.

Our casual party attitude, however, was about to change in a big hurry.

Once we were seated face to face, I began by asking him how bad his phobia was on a scale of 1 to 10, with 10 being the worst.

To my horror, the moment he went to where he needed to go in his mind in order to accurately answer such a question, he started turning a lifeless, pale color. Sweat began to bead up on his forehead and under his eyes – that fast!

I myself felt some sort of wave pass over me in a silent woosh.

I was shocked at the strength of his reaction, and how it affected me as well. In my clinic days in homeopathic college, I had seen and even successfully treated a few cases of phobia with a homeopathic remedy alone, but they were mild phobias compared to this. This was an extreme phobia, and I was about to do my very first TFT treatment in public at a poker party – yikes!

At this point, the Qi Gong instructor (let's call him Al) was clearly tuned into his phobia, and although I seriously considered changing my mind and declining to treat him in public, I decided instead that even if the treatment only worked a little bit, it would be better to provide him some relief than none at all.

So, I proceeded – a true case of the blind leading the blind.

IV

As the sweat continued to bead up, Al said rather unemotionally, "It's a **10**."

Darn nearly in a state of panic myself, I said: "OK. Now just copy me, Al, and tap here, and here, and here," I said, tapping under my own eye, and under my arm, and below my collarbone – just as they did in the video.

Al followed me exactly as we went through what I now know is the standard three point TFT algorithm for phobia and anxiety.

As soon as we had completed the entire algorithm once, I said: "OK, now what number is it?" He looked at me with a sort of disbelieving stare and said, "It's a **7**."

There came the sound of some oo-ing and aw-ing from the small crowd now gathered around watching our 'parlor trick'. I was so involved and present with Al that the sound seemed to come from somewhere off in the distance.

"Good" I said, "Let's continue then. Now tap here, and here, and here," I said, while tapping out the same phobia algorithm on my own self again, while he followed me exactly. In spite of the noise, the party, and my own fear of the possibility of having gotten into something that might be over my head, Al and I were alert, fully concentrating, and completely locked-in to what we were doing.

We continued to repeat the sequence of the same three major anxiety points followed by a series of eye and hand gestures called the "9 Gamut" series, and then we repeated the three major anxiety points again - just as in the video.

"OK" I said, once we had completed the second round, "what number is it now?"

He re-tuned his thinking to the same place he had gone to in his mind when I had first asked him, only now, it was very easy to see that he didn't feel the same level of anxiety or perturbation when thinking of the exact same problem, as he had before. It was amazing. How could a thought that had put him into a state of utter and visible panic only a moment ago, suddenly and obviously begin to lose it's tortuous hold on him by simply tapping a few spots on his body?

"It's a **5**" he said, as the guests watched in what was becoming a palpable silence, as we were all captivated and impressed by the rapid change in Al's state of being and visible reaction. He had switched from a grayish-green color to rather pinkish, and was clearly looking more relaxed as well.

"OK" I said, "Let's proceed. Tap here, here, and here," I said, taking him through the same phobia algorithm again, and once again stopping at the end of the sequence to ask what his subjective level of distress was upon thinking of his phobia now, compared to what it was when he thought about his phobia at the beginning of the treatment.

Sure enough, his level of upset had dropped yet again, just like in the video. It was down to a **3** now. I was both amazed and thrilled, trying to keep from grinning from ear to ear. I was so happy ☺.

"OK" I said, as nonchalantly as I could. "Let's continue then. Tap here, here, and here," I said, taking him through the same sequence, and ending with the same question.

"It's gone," he said, staring at me in wide-eyed disbelief. "It's gone."

"Wonderful." I said, trying to downplay the height of my internal excitement.

"Now, you need to do some things to test it out when you get home. Please call me if it comes back at all, even a little bit, OK?"

8

"OK", he said, and we returned our chairs back to the card table as if not that much had happened, although it was equally clear that something really huge had happened.

We were each grinning steadily and making that particular sort of silent acknowledging-eye-contact-cum-nod that two people often make between themselves when a significant event has occurred, transporting them both to a shared place beyond words.

V

There were a few comments and questions about the 'treatment' and then everyone returned to playing cards and enjoying the evening. In my mind, however, I was completely excited by the result and could hardly wait until Al got home to test the treatment on his own. At the time, it didn't occur to me (as it would now) to simply ask for a ladder so we could test his phobia then and there.

At some point, Al left the table along with some others in search of food. People were milling about enjoying themselves, and there was that feeling of waiting for the midnight count-down to song and celebration. The youngsters had streamers and whistles and music all ready to go.

VI

After eating some delicious East Indian food, I returned to the table for another round of cards.

In a short while, a woman whom I hadn't yet met came up to me and said: "What did you do to my husband?"

Oh my gosh, my heart nearly stopped. "Why?" I said: "Is he alright?"

"Oh, yes" she said, "he's great actually. He's downstairs dancing. This is the first time he's danced in public in over twenty years" she said. "He's got a real phobia about dancing in public. What did you do to him?"

Happily relieved, I told her we had just done a brief TFT treatment for his phobia of heights.

"Well", she said, "whatever you did, it took away his fear of dancing too!"

VII

About three weeks later, Al's wife called me requesting an appointment for a treatment for her own fear of driving over bridges.

Although Al and I had agreed he would call me if his phobia returned, I took the opportunity to ask her how Al was doing. "Let's put it this way," she said, "this Sunday, he was up on a ladder taking frozen leaves out of the eaves."

I asked her to put Al on the phone.

"What percent better is your phobia?" I asked him.

"Oh, amazing really" he said. "It's about 85 to 90% better!"

"What's different?" I asked.

"Well, I can do pretty much anything I want to do now. Like I can go up on a ladder and even climb onto the roof if I want to, whereas before, I could only go to the second step on a ladder before becoming paralyzed with fear."

"That's terrific." I said. "How come you think it's only 85-90% better? What is it you can't do?" I asked.

"Well," he said, "I don't think I could stand on that glass floor at the top of the CN Tower."

"Me neither!" I said, laughing.

We agreed that one could be phobia-free, and still not want to stand on the glass floor at the top of Toronto's CN Tower - the largest free-standing structure in the world. Although, I added, if he really wanted to, he was welcome to call me for further TFT treatment for that particular isolated fear.

VIII

Al's was my first TFT phobia case, and the result we achieved in only a couple of minutes seemed like a miracle - to both of us.

For me, the idea of being able to treat and eliminate such a severe phobia, in any amount of time, was a source of joy.

IX

In the days that followed, I was keen to re-try the poker party experiment, and actively sought out people to practice on - my children, grandchildren, friends, neighbors, and strangers - anyone I could find who had a phobia or fear they wanted eliminated.

And in every case, it worked like magic.

I was completely sold on TFT and could hardly wait to learn more.

X

In the following months and years, I completed formal training in TFT with Dr. Roger Callahan, beginning with a home study course on the theory and history of TFT, followed by a three-day class in TFT Diagnosis taught by Roger and his well respected and enthusiastic wife and CEO par excellence, Joanne Callahan. Following that, I chose six months of telephone support from Dr. Callahan, on an as-needed basis, while treating my own clients in my private practice, near Toronto.

For those who have never studied Thought Field Therapy, the training can be taken on four different levels, each inter-related. They are:

Algorithm Level (TFT-Algo)
The "Five Minute Phobia Cure" which I used to demonstrate TFT on Al at the poker party, is a perfect example of the use of TFT Algorithms. The Phobia Algorithm is that series of taps which Al did on his own body while he was thinking of his phobia. That is, while his **thought field** was tuned to the upsetting experience of his extreme fear of heights, he simultaneously tapped on a specific sequence of spots or points on his own body, until the bad feelings were gone, while thinking of the same problem.

This sequence of points, discovered and proved by Dr. Callahan to be curative in most cases of phobia, is called a TFT Phobia Algorithm. It was the first algorithm developed by Dr. Callahan, and now there are about thirty approved algorithms, all tested and proven to be 80% or more effective in thousands and thousands of cases worldwide.

A quick and easy way to learn more about the fascinating story behind Roger Callahan's discovery of TFT is by watching the "Five Minute Phobia Cure" video which has an informative introduction to TFT, or by reading one of his books called "Tapping the Healer Within".

<u>Diagnosis Level</u> (TFTdx)

This level of TFT, which involves diagnosing and treating with a specific sequence for that particular problem or condition, is called causal diagnosis and is the method used when or if a standard TFT algorithm does not eliminate the problem fully.

TFT Diagnosis is done by muscle-testing the client using the Muscle Response Test (MRT), while they hold two fingers on specific spots or points (acupuncture end-points) while thinking of their specific problem. The strength or weakness of such a muscle test indicates to the trained and sensitive practitioner, which spots need to be treated, and in what sequence, in order to eliminate that specific problem.

For example, let's say a person has a problem which they report feels like a 9 on a feel-bad scale of 1 to 10, with 10 being the worst. If for some reason treatment with an appropriate TFT algorithm did not reduce their problem enough, then TFT Diagnosis can be used to locate other specific individualized points, the treatment of which will likely bring the remainder of the problem down to a 1. And voila` - a rapid reduction of the problem.

TFT Diagnosis is basically a way of selecting a privately tailored tapping sequence from and for a person for whom an off-the-rack standard TFT algorithm (all of which were developed through TFT causal diagnosis) does not quite fit.

<u>Advanced Practitioner Level (TFT-Adv)</u>

This training consists of advanced work in TFT self-testing and self-treatment and includes Voice Technology procedures. The training provides the skills and knowledge for determining specific protocols to address a wide range of problems, including how to identify and neutralize individual energy toxins, and chronic and recurring problems on oneself, and over the telephone.

Voice Technology (TFT-VT)

This level of training is for Advanced TFT Practitioners and deals with how to test and treat others with TFT using Dr. Callahan's objective procedures while listening to their voice and checking it for various perturbations in the Thought Field, and for diagnosing the correct treatment points and sequences.

XI

During those initial years of studying TFT, I was fortunate to be able to have Dr. Callahan as my TFT therapist during a period of multiple traumatic events all occurring within a short period of time in which I lost my mother, my father, two dear friends, my 18-year-old dog, and my 17-year marriage. As if that was not enough, I was then crushed in a stampede of people running from gunfire in New Orleans, resulting in major surgeries to my shoulder and hip. Though it seemed as though luck was against me, I was nonetheless very fortunate to have Dr. Callahan and his amazing discovery of TFT to assist me through such challenging times. As my dear old Irish Nanny would have said: "Auch indeed, he was a God-sent."

XII

One night prior to a surgery, when it was too late to call Roger, I lay in bed in a considerable amount of pain and emotional distress trying desperately and unsuccessfully to treat myself with TFT algorithms. I didn't have the same skills I now have to treat myself properly with the standard TFT algorithms, and nothing I tried was working. There was no one there to test me for the correct points or procedures.

What I really needed that night was some good TFT causal diagnosis to help me with the pain and misery, but I didn't know of any way I could test my own self in order to identify the correct TFT treatment points, and most especially to test and correct my own reversals. I certainly wasn't going to call Roger in the middle of the night. This was my on-going problem.

I had heard of a few methods of self-testing and wished I knew how to get them to work on me. One such method, called the "O-ring", is done by forming an "O" with the thumb and tiny finger of one hand, and trying to open that closed "O" by inserting a held-together thumb and index finger of the other hand into the closed "O" and attempt to force it open by opening up the inserted thumb and index finger against the "O-ring" to see if it opens. If it can be opened, it indicates weakness, and if it cannot be opened it indicates strength. I couldn't get the "O-ring" method to work with any sort of consistent results. I would test something quite simple twice in a row such as "My name is Norma" vs. "My name is Fred", and I'd get a different response each time. Clearly, this test wasn't working for me and couldn't be trusted to give a reliable result - at least not then.

I lay there thinking about muscle-testing in general and how great it would be if there was a truly reliable way to self-muscle-test such that you could treat your own self with TFT in the middle of the night. This was something that was wanted and needed by a lot more people than just me, I thought. I couldn't stop thinking about it.

XIII

I began fantasy-designing various sorts of mechanisms and machines that I thought might function as reliable self-muscle-testers. Each was based on the traditional Applied Kinesiology method of muscle-testing as developed by chiropractor George Goodheart in 1964, and included the basic idea of pressing down on a person's out-stretched arm. Only in this case, the various contraptions I imagined allowed you to press down on a mildly-flexible horizontal bar which was attached to a vertical post, and which, as you pressed down on the rod, would move downwards, or not. The amount of movement would indicate on a gauge or dial the degree of strength or weakness in the force you needed to exert to cause the rod to move. Hence, indicating a weak or strong response.

It seemed like a great idea to me, and still does. It was not, however, something that could be developed over night, and I needed something I could use *now*. I was determined to keep my mind on it until I came up with a way to self-test myself that very night.

By now, it was nearing 4 a.m.

How about a bathroom scale I wondered? Maybe you could push down on a scale instead of a bar and get a good difference in pressure on a standard TFT muscle test.

I hobbled into the bathroom and put my digital scale up on the counter in order to check it out. I decided to test myself (without making the usual TFT corrections first) by simply thinking of something really good (this test works best when tuned to an event or feeling involving yourself in which you felt really good), and then pressing down on the scale with my left hand. The reading began at 20.5 and settled at 18.5. Then, I thought of something really bad involving myself and causing me to feel badly. The reading began at 20.5 and stopped at 17.5.   Not much of a difference – one pound, but worth trying again in case there proved to be a consistent difference. I tried it over and over using various TFT protocols, and although there was usually a noticeable difference between weak and strong reactions, it was inconsistent, unreliable, tiring, and basically sloppy. One minute I tested strong for "Norma", and the next minute I tested strong for "Fred". ☺

I guess 'sloppy', was how I had felt about muscle-testing in general. In homeopathic college, we had been taught to use the standard Muscle Response Test (MRT) to determine food sensitivities in a client, and although I could see how it might be useful if it could be trusted, I never really trusted it because it never seemed to give consistent results. As well, I had had several experiences in which practitioners had attempted, either by over or under-pressing on my arm to prove a point they had pre-decided upon, and then went about maneuvering my poor arm into agreeing with them. In fact, one practitioner pushed so hard on my strong arm that it caused a visible struggle, which ended with him saying, "See, I told you it would be weak!"

Nonetheless, intellectually and experientially, I knew that something was definitely happening in a person whose arm one moment was normally strong, and then a moment later, simply by thinking of something negative, or being exposed to a toxin, that same arm was suddenly and demonstrably weak. I had seen several clients who were actually unable to hold their arm up when tuning to a distressing thought. That is, their out-stretched arm would drop all by itself when changing their thought from a positive to a negative feeling. So, something was going on. The question was: what was going on, and how to use that information in a way that could be trusted for diagnostic muscle-testing.

It wasn't until I learned about Roger Callahan's brilliant discovery of TFT and Psychological Reversal that I became interested in reconsidering the value of muscle-testing. TFT in general and Psychological Reversal (PR) especially, take muscle-testing and elevate it with a higher degree of accuracy, making it more reliable than it can be without the knowledge of Psychological Reversal and some of the other TFT protocols, because with these specific protocols, one is able to identify and correct both the tester and the testee for the presence of various PRs, at any point in a therapeutic session. TFT and the identification of and correction of PR take the much disputed and often doubtful results of the standard muscle-test and turn the method into a force to be reckoned with. The correction of PR moves muscle-testing out of the realm of inconsistent and irregular and into the realm of reliable and accurate.

For example, with the standard two-person muscle-test known as MRT, when a person is being tested for a reaction to a particular substance such as sugar (to find out whether they test weak or strong to it), the client holds a cube of sugar or a vial containing sugar or an extract of sugar (or simply says the word 'sugar' and hence is thinking about sugar) while the tester performs the standard muscle response test (MRT) on the client's out-stretched arm. If the arm tests weak, it would appear that the client is showing some reactive effect from the essence of or mere thought of sugar, and is therefore exhibiting a sensitivity reaction to sugar, or the idea of sugar, in some regard. That is, in the presence of sugar (or some other challenge) the client loses a noticeable measure of their normal physical strength which was present "in the clear" only a moment before, when they were not thinking of sugar.

If, however, the client can maintain normal before-test strength, and their outstretched arm remains strong when challenged with sugar, it is assumed in standard muscle-testing, that the client is therefore not negatively affected by sugar, and the test for sugar is ended there, with the resulting strong test assumed to mean that the client is OK with sugar. That's how a basic MRT is carried out and interpreted.

In general, the basic MRT has its merits of course, because a weak test is most often indicative of some sort of sensitivity provided that (and here's the important difference brought to light by TFT) neither the tester nor the client has a PR during the muscle-testing procedure. That is, with the standard MRT, if you test weak for sugar, you can trust that sugar makes you weak, as long as neither you nor the tester are under the influence of a Psychological Reversal (PR). If you or the person testing you is psychologically reversed then you cannot trust the test result until all PR's are identified and corrected with simple TFT procedures and the test then re-done for accuracy.

Hence, as a result of Roger Callahan's discovery of PR, the TFT muscle-testing procedure is done differently than the standard MRT. The TFT muscle-test is more complex, revealing, and offers more reliable results, which, following from the above example, are as follows:

1) <u>If a person tests weak</u> for sugar on the initial test, that weakness can be instantly corrected with a TFT toxin procedure such that the person is then relieved of the weakening effect of the sugar test and able to maintain strength when re-tested for sugar. And although sugar should be avoided by the sensitive person, the major difference here is that if sugar is ingested in the future, accidentally or purposely, the effects of it can be neutralized with specific TFT toxin procedures. Any related physical or emotional symptoms can be relieved on the spot. If there is any question as to whether the tester may be suffering from PR and hence affecting the test, then this phenomenon can also be checked, corrected, and the test re-done for increased accuracy.

2) <u>If a person tests strong</u> for sugar on the initial test, this reaction, although good, is not automatically assumed to be trustworthy until two other tests are performed, the results of which determine whether the first test is reliable or not, by making sure that the client is not **'reversed'** (TFT jargon for **PR**) prior to the test and/or has not suddenly become 'reversed' by the substance or by the name of the substance, and also whether the practitioner is 'reversed' or not, which in the regular style of two-person muscle testing, can very much effect the test results in ways unknown to either person.

More simply put, if you apply the correct TFT protocols (to follow) during a standard two-person muscle-test, or during a reliable self-muscle-test, you get a more accurate result than if you muscle-test without using TFT procedures to identify and correct for various forms of Psychological Reversal.

XIV

Back to that night, and the following days... .

The idea of pushing down on a scale or some such mechanism was a nice try, but too unreliable and too complicated as well, because it would require some sort of dial for taking the readings. There had to be another way. What if you could test by lifting something up, I wondered, even though it was the opposite motion of pushing something down. Would that work?

I went downstairs to get the 5-pound weight sitting next to my exercise video and looked around for something that was shoulder height. I put the weight on the fireplace mantle and stood with my arm held straight out to the side, holding the weight in my hand. Then I proceeded to test myself by first thinking of something really good and then lifting the weight.

My arm and the weight went straight up into the air like a feather. This might work, I thought. I got myself ready for the second half of the test by thinking of something bad (like my aching hip which I learned much later had been fractured in the stampede) and then lifting the weight with my left and un-injured arm. The weight felt heavier, yet still went up into the air. Too bad, I thought - the weight was too light. In fact, the weight was so much too light that it seemed I'd probably have to use a weight far too heavy to be appropriate for this idea to actually work. Feeling somewhat pre-defeated, I went back to my bed for some warmth. I lay there pondering.

I thought of the stories I'd heard about Edison and the light bulb, and others who had kept on trying when they felt defeated, in spite of tremendous odds, until they eventually succeeded. So I decided that if I was really serious about this weight-lifting idea, there was no use throwing in the towel until I had tried it with a weight that was actually heavy enough to get a response in the negative thought field. And even if such a weight would be too heavy for practical use, it was worth taking it to that point to find out, rather than giving up without actually knowing.

XV

There was a little garden shed in my back yard, and I thought I had one or two heavy chrome weights rusting away out there. I went downstairs and threw my winter coat on over my nightgown and went out into the blustery cold and pre-dawn bleakness of my back yard to look for the weights, thinking: "This better work!"

I found two 10 and one 12-pound weight. Because of my injuries it took me two trips to carry one of each size back over the frozen 'tundra' of my wintry world.

Once I had the weights in the house I decided I needed to test myself sitting down. I was too tired and sore to keep standing in front of the mantle.

I took the 10-pound weight upstairs and put it on the bathroom counter. I got the little step-stool I kept in my closet and set it up in front of the bathroom counter - perfect height.

I sat down sideways to the counter with my feet on the bottom step and my left arm stretched out toward the weight and took hold of it with my left hand. Here's a picture of one of my grandsons modeling it for you:

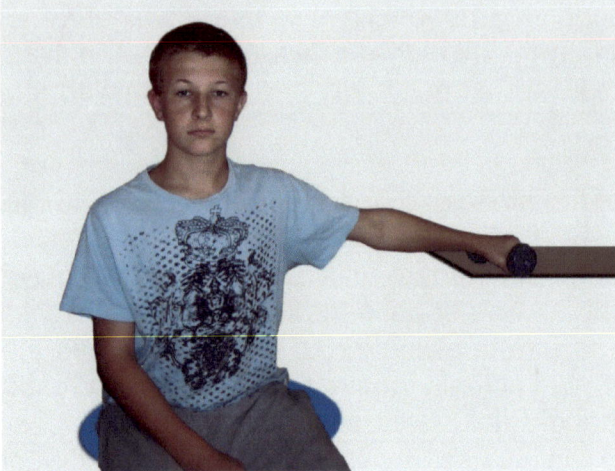

Once again, I thought of something really good (like lying in the sun on the hot rocks of Ontario's beautiful northland and feeling completely happy). Then I lifted the weight. It came up, though it was definitely heavier than the 5-pound weight. I put it down and got ready for the second half of the test by thinking of something that made me feel badly (a past betrayal), and again lifted the weight. What a difference! This time, it felt so heavy I could barely lift it more than an inch or so off the counter. It wouldn't go any higher with all my strength. This was getting exciting, though it seemed I needed an even heavier weight. I went downstairs to get the 12-pound weight.

XVI

With the 12-pound weight in hand, I once again thought of something really good and lifted the weight. It was heavy for sure, yet came up about a foot, with some strain. Then I thought of something bad and lifted the weight again. I couldn't budge it.
I tried it again, first thinking of something good, and lifting it up about a foot. And then thinking of something bad and lifting it up.

I couldn't move it…not even a tiny bit. It was as though the weight was glued to the counter top - completely stuck there. This is it, I thought. This can work!

By now it was well past dawn, but rather than being tired from being up all night, I was wide awake. Although I was still in considerable physical pain, I intended to keep going and keep testing.

XVII

I began with the standard TFT test for PR which uses the phrase "I want to be healthy", and then it's opposite, the phrase "I want to be sick". The first phrase tested strong – that is, I could lift the weight easily. The second phrase tested weak – that is, I could not lift the weight at all. Amazing really! I went on to test all the standard TFT phrases for the various levels of Psychological Reversal, which you will find laid out for you in the SELF-TESTING CHART on page 40. This was what I had hoped and prayed for.

XVIII

By then my left arm was getting tired, so I turned my stool to face the counter and the weight. I began to test myself with both hands holding the weight, both arms outstretched in front of me, my two hands side by side on the weight. Like this:

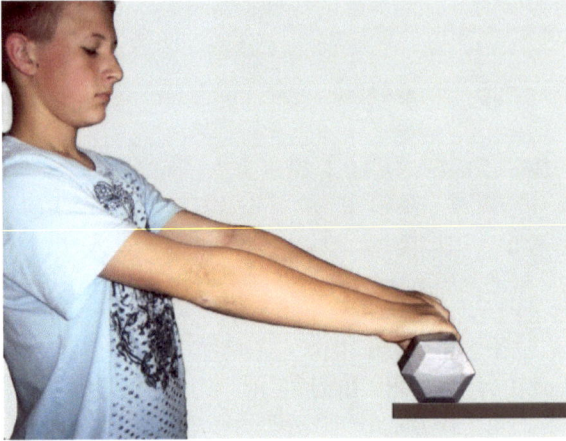

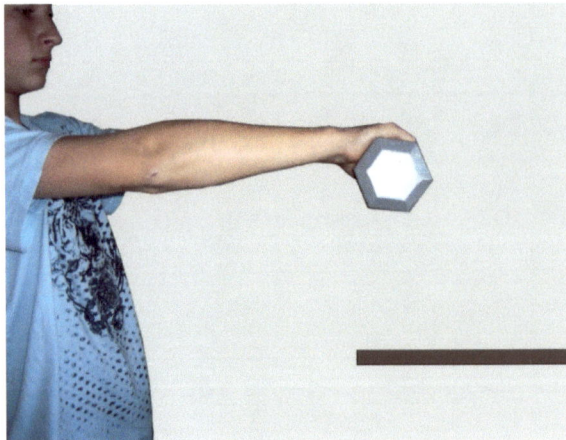

Amazingly, this method of using both arms to lift a heavier weight worked equally well, though as I now know, the 12-pound weight was far too heavy for me. A heavier weight was necessary at the beginning, however, in order for me to be able to feel the subtle though exacting difference there is between a weak or strong muscle response. That is, to be able to recognize, locate, and feel that internal tipping point that makes lifting a weight vary from relative ease in lifting (that is, not requiring all of one's strength by any means), to absolute temporary impossibility (that is, not budging at all, even when using every bit of one's strength in attempting to lift the exact same weight).

The key to perfection in learning and using the NRG Method of self-muscle-testing is **using your regular strength at each and every attempt to lift the weight**. That way, you are able to focus on the test, rather than on the result, because you can either lift the weight, or you cannot. If, during self-testing and using the correct TFT phrases, you are unable to lift a small weight which you could easily lift only a moment ago, then something is happening to prevent you from doing so. And that something, when properly identified, is in TFT called a Psychological Reversal, and referred to by thousands of TFT'ers around the world, as simply **"PR"** or being **"reversed"**.

This ability to use one's regular or full strength during self-muscle-testing is something that cannot be done during the standard two-person muscle-test without causing one or the other of the two people some sort of pain, harm, battle of strength, or test confusion. Neither can full strength be used in the O-ring method, because two fingers of one hand are testing two fingers of the other hand and both hands belong to the tester. In self-muscle-testing with the NRG Method, however, using one's regular strength is the key to success. It allows you to trust the test completely, because the weight is an inanimate object without a point of view. You can either lift the weight, or you can't.

Accurate self-muscle-testing accomplishes many things and has far-reaching implications:

*it removes the common doubt or suspicion that often accompanies the standard two-person muscle response test (MRT) that the tester is pushing too hard or too lightly on the client's arm and hence influencing the test in some way;

*it eliminates the need for an outside tester;

*it provides privacy and convenience for self-testing and self-treating of personal issues at home, including issues that one might never reveal, even to a therapist;

*it can be used by practitioners while surrogating for others without having to touch the client;

*it can be used by clients on themselves in the presence of their practitioner, eliminating the need for the practitioner to use the MRT or to touch the client;

*it can be used by clients and practitioners on themselves in the privacy of their own home, for the identification and TFT treatment of various PR's, toxins, and the use of TFT Algorithms;

*it can be used for self-causal-diagnosis. Once a person or client has learned TFTdx *and* **the NRG Method**, they become a trained TFT practitioner doing self-treatment with TFT causal diagnosis;

*it can be used with other therapies or modalities that use MRT;

*it is completely portable and can be used anywhere, anytime. When without a gym weight, you can use a filled water bottle, a book, or anything that is the right weight for you…a hefty rock, or, how about an Oscar!

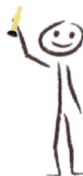

CHOOSING THE RIGHT SIZE WEIGHT FOR YOU

When first learning this method, **you will need to have a selection of a few different sized weights available,** until you know which weight is the right size for you personally. Sorting this out takes only a short time (varies per person), and once you have it sorted out, you'll need only one weight that works best for you.

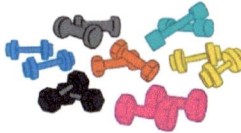

Over time, you'll be able to reduce the original starting weight to an ever lower weight as you become more sensitive to your own muscle responses.

Generally speaking, to begin with, it's best to start with a weight that is relatively heavy to lift with one arm, which for most people (male and female) will probably be a 5,10, or 12 pound weight to begin with. I currently use a two-pound weight for my personal testing, though I needed a much heavier weight (12 lbs) before I got my first accurate self-muscle-test response. It took a fairly heavy weight for me to prove to myself that the method was indeed reliable.

I have taught this method to people who have been able to use a 1 or 2 pound weight right from the start, and others who needed to use 15 pounds or more before they could get a reliable first test. I once demonstrated this method to a muscle-bound gym equipment salesman who prided himself on his physical strength and said there was no way that anything could ever make him be unable to lift such a small amount of weight. I started him with 30 pounds, using both arms held out in front of him. He thought of something good, and lifted the weight, and then he thought of something bad and the weight didn't budge. The sudden inability to lift the weight frightened him. He jumped up off the chair and said I must be a witch. He didn't understand that the momentary weakness was real, was in his own body, and had nothing to do with me.

The point is that with the right weight you will get an accurate test response, so be sure to take the time to gather a few weights so you will have plenty of options for a successful start. It's temporary that you need more than one or two weights, so perhaps you could borrow some from a friend, or sign out a few from a local gym. I had one client who used various size drinking bottles and filled them each with different amounts of stones and water, and weighed and labeled them.

Now that you have a selection of weights to choose from, here's what to do: choose your weight and self-muscle-test from a sitting or a standing position, with your outstretched arm comfortable and properly placed to mimic the position of a standard two-person muscle-test. The difference is that when you are self-muscle-testing with **the NRG method**, rather than having someone else press down on your outstretched arm to demonstrate your strength or weakness, you will be *lifting* the weight to indicate your own strength or weakness. Simply put, **when you can lift the weight the test is strong, and when you cannot lift the weight the test is weak.**

28

INSTRUCTIONS FOR CHOOSING THE CORRECT WEIGHT:

Place a chair next to a table, ledge, or any flat surface that allows you to sit with your arm outstretched to the side, resting on the table, about a foot lower than shoulder height. With the weight in hand, you will be lifting your arm upward to shoulder height. You can be sitting or standing.

Sit on the chair with your body facing forward, and your left arm extended straight out from your left side, resting on the table. Like this:

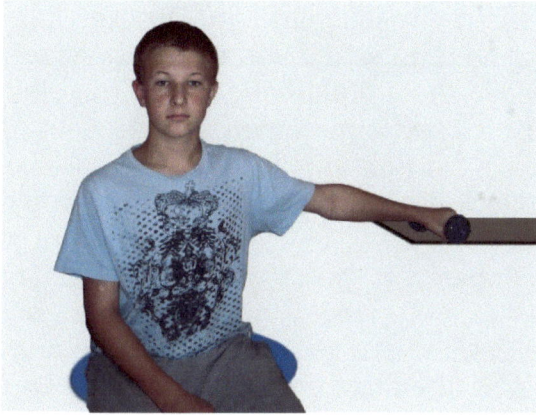

Or, you can stand if you prefer. Like this:

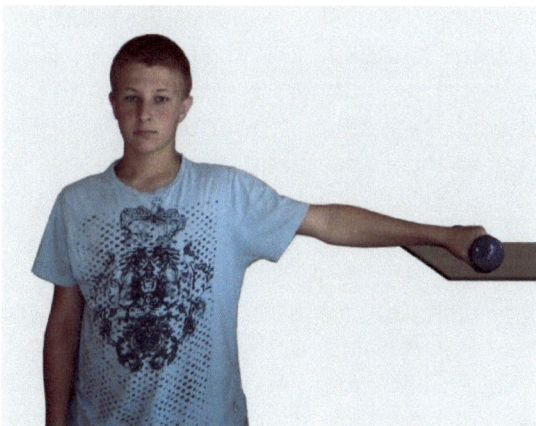

First, pick a weight that you think is suitable for you: 5, 8, or 10 pounds. If you are a very sensitive person, or physically weak, you may be able to start with a 3-pound weight right away. Most people, however, need to start with a slightly heavier weight until they "get it", and then they can reduce it to a lower and lower weight as they become more sensitive to the physical response within their own body.

Ready? Sit relaxed and place your left hand on the weight, as though you were going to lift it...and keep reading these instructions:

Although either arm will do just fine for self-muscle-testing, I recommend the left arm whenever possible, because that's what John Diamond, the grandfather of muscle-testing, first recommended be used - perhaps because using the left hand implies accessing the right brain (?). In any case, either arm will work for self-muscle-testing - and use your left arm if you can.

Now that you have your hand on the weight, you are simply going to lift the weight straight up, about a foot or so, to where your arm is level with your shoulder. For now, you are lifting the weight to see how it feels to you - that it feels a comfortable size for you. That is, it feels slightly heavy, though certainly not uncomfortable to lift, and also is not too light either - you want to feel some resistance or heaviness when you lift it, because it's a mild muscle-challenge test. If it's uncomfortable or too heavy to lift up readily, then choose a lighter weight and try it again. Likewise, if it feels as light as a feather, then pick a slightly heavier weight and try again. If needed, try different sizes, until you have a weight that you think is a good test weight for you and your arm.

Now that you've chosen a starting weight, we're going to do a couple of preliminary tests to see if this is the correct weight for you. You're going to be lifting the weight again, but this time, before you lift it, you're going to first **tune your thought field (TF)** to something positive that makes you feel good when thinking of it now. This thought/image/sound/feeling can be a happy memory from the past, or a delightful expectation for the future, as long as it makes you feel good when thinking about it now.

For simplicity's sake when doing this test, I often **tune** my **TF** to how content and happy I feel on a hot and breezy summer's day, relaxing on the warm granite rocks of Ontario's cottage country, with the sound of the shining water lapping against the shoreline, and that old sun soft and warm against my skin, and the clean buoyant smell of the freshest air.

Any memory that gives you a solid positive feeling will do. You can have fun recalling a time when you burst out laughing, or had a feeling of exhilaration after a physical (or romantic) work-out ☺, or any successful, fun, fulfilling, or joyful experience. If you can't think of one readily, then imagine one.

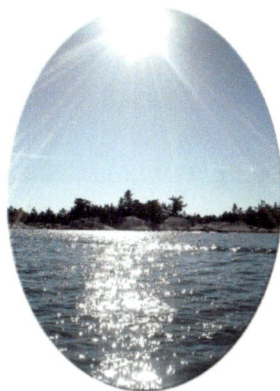

Once you've tuned your thought field **(TF)** to a good feeling, you can go ahead and lift the weight up off the table and then set it down again right away. It is not a strength test per se, it's a test to see how the weight feels when your **TF** is positively tuned. That's all it is for now - a test to see how the weight feels to you.

So far, you've lifted the weight twice. Once while thinking of nothing, which is called testing "in the clear", and once while tuning your thought field to a positive memory or thought. It is likely that the weight came up fairly easily both times. If the weight seemed too heavy for your arm, however, then you need to re-do the test with a lighter weight. And if the weight seemed too light to offer any firmness or comfortable resistance, then you need to try a slightly heavier weight.

Now that you have a sense of how the weight feels when you are positively tuned (perhaps it feels slightly lighter than when you tested it "in the clear"), you are going to do the corresponding half of that same test. That is, this time you are going to momentarily tune your **TF** to a negative memory from the past, or an expectation of something negative in the future, and then test yourself in that **thought field**.

This tuning of your **TF** to something that made you feel badly, is also for you to feel the difference between how your muscles respond when you think of something bad, as compared with how they respond when you think of something good. Both tests are done *exactly* the same, only the thought content is different.

Keep this test easy and simple like the first test, and choose a mildly negative memory from the past that made you feel badly - not a traumatic memory, and don't dwell on it. Just think of it for a second and test. You don't want to get upset or overly-reactive, you just want to see how your muscles respond when you think a negative thought, such as a time when your feelings were hurt, or you felt upset about something or someone.

Now, with your **TF** re-tuned to something that makes you feel negatively when you think of it now, you can go ahead and lift the weight again, using the same natural strength you used when you lifted it while you were thinking of something that made you feel good. **That's the trick - to always use the same natural strength to lift the weight.** Use your natural strength every time, the way you would do if you were lifting any other object - a book, a bottle, a purse. Just lift it, and then set it down.

One of three things will occur when you lift the weight in a negative TF:

1) the weight stays put and does not move;
2) the weight moves but only a little and feels inordinately heavy;
3) the weight comes up off the table.

Interpretation of the three results:

1) If the weight stays put and doesn't move, you have a perfect test response for this situation of thinking of something bad. That is, your muscles have become momentarily weak and you cannot lift the weight while you

are in this negative **TF**, even though you would be able to lift the exact same weight quite easily if you were tuning your **TF** to a positive thought, or not thinking.

2) If the weight moves up only a bit and feels inordinately heavy, or only comes up at one end, you need to re-do the test with the same weight, to see if you get a clearer response the second time. Be sure to re-tune your **TF** with a clear focus, and not be thinking of other things (including the test) while doing the test - think only of what your **TF** is tuned to, since that's what you're testing. Then, re-do the test in both the positive and the negative **TFs** again.

If the weight still moves, but only a little, you need to increase the size by one or two pounds, and this will likely give you a firmer response, and the weight will come up when you are positively tuned, and will stay put (not move) when you are negatively tuned, which is the exact response you want. But you want this clear response to come from you **using the correct weight**, and doing nothing other than tuning your **TF** and lifting the weight with your normal strength.

3) If the weight comes up off the table with little or no difference in either the positive or negative **TF,** then re-do the test again with a heavier weight until you arrive at a weight that comes up when you are in a positive **TF** and stays put (does not come up) when you are in a negative **TF**. Keep increasing the weight until you get a clear and correct response to both the positive and negative thoughts.

If, after following the directions in the above 3 options, you still test strong or weak on both the positive and negative **TFs**, then you are experiencing what is casually referred to in TFT as being "**reversed**". That is, you are testing the opposite of what is expected, normal, or healthy - you are testing strong when thinking of something bad, or testing weak when thinking of something good. If that is the case, you're in luck, because in this method, there is an easy solution. You will need to follow a very important yet simple procedure for correcting this condition, which in TFT is formally called **Psychological Reversal** (**PR**), and is one of the most brilliant of the many **TFT** discoveries of Roger Callahan, Ph.D.

The condition of "**Psychological Reversal**", when identified and correctly treated (or **un-**reversed you might say) using a simple TFT procedure, can create a rapid, noticeable and remarkable change for the better, not only in distressing psychological states, but also in many physical and emotional conditions as well. For more in depth information on this important discovery, please see Roger Callahan's books: "Stop the Nightmares of Trauma" and "Tapping the Healer Within".

In the meantime, whenever you find yourself saying things opposite to what you intended to say, such as saying "south" when you mean "north", it is caused by a Psychological Reversal (**PR**). Or, when you find that you are somehow 'shooting yourself in the foot' in your everyday dealings in life; or, you find yourself stuck in any kind of dysfunctional relationship; or, you do things contrary to what it is that you say you want to do. All of these actions are instances of **PR,** and the sooner this **state of reversal** gets corrected the better, because not only can it interfere with your ability to do something simple like choosing the right weight for learning how to accurately self-muscle-test, it can and does interfere with everything else as well, though unless we've studied TFT we're most often unaware of it.

PR is responsible not only for us saying the wrong words, and writing letters backwards, but also behind many an error in judgment regarding important actions and life choices - and most of all, **PR blocks healing**.

With this method and this knowledge, not only are you going to be aware of your own **reversals**, you are also going to be able to self-test for them and correct them. The result can be self-healing and life-altering.

Choosing the right weight, cont'd...
We didn't talk about what to do if (and this would be rare) the weight stays put and doesn't come up off the table when you're thinking of something good. Well, that too would be a **reversal** or

PR, and would require the same correction as any basic **Psychological Reversal**, which I'm going to show you now.

HOW TO CORRECT FOR PSYCHOLOGICAL REVERSAL:

It's simple - you take 2 fingers of one hand and tap the side of your other hand 15 to 20 times, right on the spot you would be using if you were karate-chopping a board. That's it!

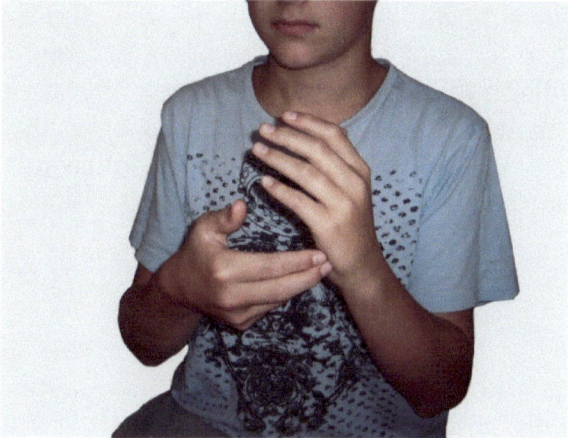

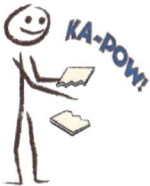

CHOOSING THE RIGHT WEIGHT FOR YOU:

Let's say you tested strong for the positive-thought test, and the weight came up and felt fine. But then, when you test for the negative thought, the weight also comes up. Well, that's kind of backwards, right? Your muscles should test strong when you're thinking something positive and weak when you're thinking something negative – it's a normal response.

If it should ever happen that you test the opposite or the reverse of what is expected or correct, then it's time to tap the side of your hand on the **PR** (karate) spot. Tap that **PR** spot 15 - 20 times, and then re-test yourself with the weight, while thinking of something good, and then while thinking of something bad.

That should be all you need to do at this stage, to choose the right weight for yourself.

Before continuing, be sure to use the information above and work with different size weights until you have a weight that comes up easily on the positive-thought test, and will not budge on the negative-thought test. That's the right weight for you, for now. It may take a few minutes or more to sort this out, but make sure you work with the weights until you have this part **100%** correct. Then you can proceed with confidence to test yourself for anything and everything you ever wanted to know.

XIX

That reminds me of the first time I showed this method to anyone. It was the day after I discovered that, if done correctly, this method is 100% dependable, and could therefore be used to accurately self-muscle-test.

I was so excited about it that I began trying it on everything and everyone. The very first person was my little grandson who walked to my house after school that day. He was in second grade. (My Grandchildren call me "Ga".)

I took him over to the ledge of my china cabinet (it looked the right height for his arm while standing up) and I put a green 5 pound weight on the ledge, and positioned him correctly. I told him I wanted to show him something – and that's all I said. Then, I had him think of something good and lift the weight up, which he did, and then said: "Ya, so...?" And then I had him think of something bad and lift the weight up, and he couldn't move it, not at all.

"Oh my gosh, Ga!" he said, "how does it do that?"

I told him that our body is all one piece and when we think of good things our muscles feel strong and when we think of bad things they feel momentarily weak, only we don't notice it because we aren't usually looking for it in this way.

You could see his little mind working away. "Try it again!" he insisted.

So I had him say "I am a boy", and the weight came up. Then say, "I am a girl", which made him giggle, and he couldn't move the weight no matter how hard he tried. "Do it again!" he said. So we did some more phrases.

"Oh my gosh, Ga," he said again, "do you know that with *this* you can find out anything you want to know?"

"Yes" I said, "almost anything."

It was one of my happier moments in life. ☺

XX

Speaking of the ability to know things, reminds me of the man who wanted to know all there was to know.

When we left off, the old monk had opened the door and said: *"Come in," and the man stooped to enter the ancient stone monastery. The heavy wooden door, blackened by age, closed with a thud. The old monk led the man down a damp stony corridor, with wooden doors on either side, to a door at the end, on the right.*

The monk opened the door, and the man entered the room.

The room was made of stone, and though bare of decoration, there were stacks upon stacks of dusty old volumes rising like stalagmites, nearly filling the room.

Other than the books, there was a wooden bed, a desk, a chair, and a tall candle.

"You can stay here," said the old monk. And with that, he left, closing the door behind him.

The man began to read the books, studying diligently day after day, week after week - living simply and working hard, as one would in an ancient monastery.

After several weeks, the old Master came into his room, carrying his staff.

"Now," said the master, "do you know everything there is to know?"

"No," said the man. "I do not."

At which point the master raised his staff and began beating the man about the head and shoulders...and then he left, closing the door behind him.

The man determined to study even harder. He went back to reading and studying and often working through the night, week in and week out.

After a few more weeks, the Master came into his room again.

"Now," he said: "do you know everything there is to know?"

"No, Master," said the man, "I do not." At which point the Master raised his staff and began beating the man about the head and shoulders...and then left.

This went on for months and months...but before we finish our story, we need to finish learning how to self-test and self-treat with the weights, using the **NRG Method** and some **TFT protocols**.

XXI

SELF-TESTING AND SELF-TREATING WITH THE WEIGHTS

Now that you have a weight that tests properly (**with 100% certainty**) for a positive and negative thought, and muscles that respond normally to a positive and negative thought, we are going to get to work on some self-testing and correcting techniques.

The first thing you're going to do is learn to identify another sort of reversal. In TFT, this one is called a "Massive Reversal" and occurs in most domains of the Thought Field when there is a reversal in your body's polarity. It's more like an electrical problem than a psychological problem per se. And in fact, this sort of reversal can be measured with a voltmeter. (see Roger Callahan's work on "Voltmeter and Psychological Reversal".)

HOW TO TEST AND CORRECT MASSIVE REVERSAL:
This PR test has 2 simple moves: **palm up/palm down.**

Sit or stand comfortably, with one hand holding the weight on the table (or ledge) as usual, and **the other hand held, palm downward, about 2" over your head,** as if you were holding a baseball cap on your head. You then lift the weight with one hand while holding the other hand palm down over your head – the weight should come up in this position, with your hand palm down over your head. Then, you flip that same hand upside down over your head so that the back of your hand is facing your head (which affects the polarity), and test again - the test should be a weak test in this position, and the weight stay put.

TFT Twins testing for PR

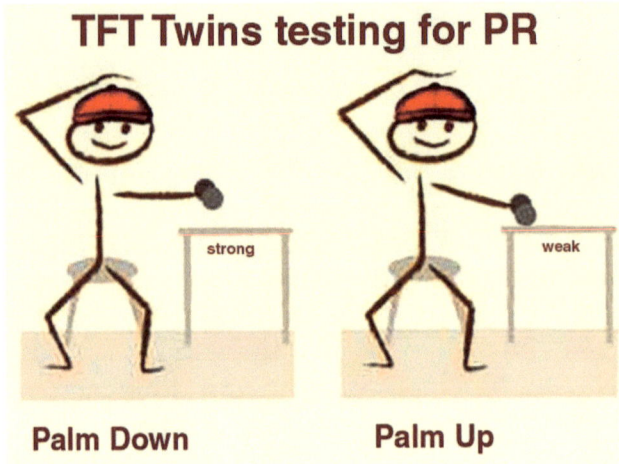

Palm Down   Palm Up

If the test is 'reversed' in any way (that is, palm down is weak instead of strong, or palm up is strong instead of weak) then you must do a simple **PR correction** which again, is also done by tapping the side of your hand on the **PR spot**.

After you tap the side of your hand about 15-20 taps, you then re-test to make sure it's testing correctly, repeating the correction if needed, until it does.

Once Massive Reversal is corrected, you can proceed with some standard TFT testing and correcting protocols.

Finally, some accurate self-testing you can trust with all your strength – phew. ☺

SELF-TESTING WITH THE NRG METHOD
AND SELF-TREATING WITH TFT REVERSAL CORRECTIONS

Begin every self-testing session the same way:

FIRST, CHECK YOURSELF FOR MASSIVE REVERSAL:
HOLD HAND OVER HEAD PALM DOWN = STRONG
HOLD HAND OVER HEAD PALM UP = WEAK
IF EITHER IS REVERSED, TAP SIDE OF HAND
then RETEST and re-treat if needed, until
corrected.

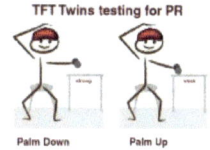
TFT Twins testing for PR
Palm Down   Palm Up

SECOND, CHECK FOR SPECIFIC REVERSAL USING THE FOLLOWING PHRASES:

1) CHECK FOR SPECIFIC REVERSAL in the PRESENT TENSE:

I WANT TO BE HEALTHY = strong
I WANT TO BE SICK = weak
I WANT TO BE COMPLETELY HEALTHY = strong
I WANT TO BE SICK = weak

IF REVERSED on any present tense phrases,
TAP SIDE OF HAND to correct -
then RETEST and re-treat if needed, until corrected.

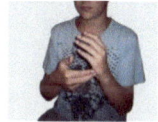

2) CHECK FOR SPECIFIC REVERSAL in the FUTURE TENSE:

I WILL BE HEALTHY = strong
I WILL BE SICK = weak
I WILL BE COMPLETELY HEALTHY = strong
I WILL BE SICK = weak

IF REVERSED on any future tense phrases
correct by TAPPING UNDER your NOSE.
then RETEST and re-treat if needed, until corrected.

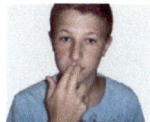

Occasionally, someone will say to me, "What if a reversal won't correct?" And my answer is, "In my experience, every reversal is correctable, though some can be more stubborn than others, and require more effort or expertise to resolve."

You have to go with what is, without letting the test itself affect your thinking one way or another. It's similar to being objective, with the added subtlety of holding a clear mind *and* keeping yourself out of the way at the same time. You are, after all, testing your own **thought field** which extends beyond your thinking and beyond your physicality. Emotions impact the thought field. Self-testing works best if you can keep a steady clear mind during testing procedures, although feeling and expressing emotions is fine, even desirable, during self-treatment.

If any sort of reversal is not correcting easily, try taking a break and drinking a couple of glasses of good filtered water, and then resume treatment beginning with the massive reversal test again – this is often all that is needed.

Be patient, and keep your thought field free of negative focus, because doing this correctly rather than quickly, is what is important, and what will give you the highest degree of success in self-treatment.

The goal is to **master this self-muscle-testing method 100%** so that you can use it with confidence, and proceed to self-test and self-treat at a really deep level, such that you become healthier and happier in every way you can think of, and in all directions of time.

Now, having said all of the above, we need to address what to do in the rare case that you run into a reversal that refuses to correct. If you have not been formally trained in TFT, you may not be aware of reversals that are caused by toxins. Or, you may be aware of them because you have felt badly or had symptoms after eating or smelling certain things such as milk or perfume.

In such a case, it's wise to identify the toxin and remove it. Now that you know how to self-muscle-test, you may want to study TFT in more depth so that you can learn to test and treat yourself for the effects of what in TFT are called Individual Energy Toxins (I.E.T.s), such as wheat, dairy, corn, perfume, personal products and supplements, etc. In TFT, there's a simple and effective toxin treatment that can assist you in identifying and eliminating the ill-effects of those things you may be sensitive to and which may be causing chronic reversals and other correctable problems. This method is easy to learn and easy to do, and the treatment and removal of toxins, as well as traumas, is a way to correct the most stubborn reversals.

In the meantime, if needed, you can call any number of Advanced TFT Practitioners (including myself at www.NRGHolistic.com) to assist you in correcting a stubborn reversal quickly. TFT Practitioner contact information can be found at the ATFT website.

If you'd like to read some remarkable case histories gathered from TFT practitioners around the world (including several of my cases), please see "Tapping the Body's Energy Pathways" by Roger & Joanne Callahan.

ONCE YOU HAVE CORRECTED BASIC REVERSALS:

The first thing to do, either before or after correcting your basic reversals, is to decide what it is you'd like to test, correct, or treat. For example, when I first developed this method, I made a list of all the things I wanted to work on, and then spent hours working on them, one by one.

Modeling my initial self-testing statements after the standard TFT phrases: "I want to be healthy/I want to be sick", I was so thrilled to finally be able to test myself, I went at it full bore with the intent of clearing up anything and everything I could possibly find in my thought field - a huge spring cleaning of my psyche, you might say. I began by checking all sorts of emotional states that I was aware of, as well as those I could be unaware of, to see if there were any reversals lurking around in there, and to correct them. Needless to say, I cried and laughed and yawned…a lot. It was an amazing process, and the liberation of being able to treat myself, and in complete privacy, was exhilarating.

I'm not sure why it happens, but there's something about doing cathartic work with TFT that causes yawning - in me, and in most of my clients too. Yawning that is quickly followed by increased alertness, rather than the sort of yawning that signals tiredness.

To create your own self-treatment plan, search within and make your own list of things to check and correct that are reflective of your life's issues and emotional themes. Here are a few of the things I tested and corrected myself for at the start, though they are only a small portion of what I did, over time:

I want to be strong/I want to be weak
I am strong/I am weak
I want to be happy/I want to be sad
I am happy/I am sad
I am OK
I love myself/I hate myself
I am worthy/I am unworthy
I am worthy/I am worthless
I forgive myself/I judge myself
I forgive myself/I blame myself
I want to live/I want to die…and so on.

I did hours of this sort of self-testing for reversals. My list was about 3 pages long. I also tested each phrase in both the present and future tenses, just as we do when testing and correcting basic reversals in TFT, except that my data-searching personal test phrases were not part of standard TFT protocol.

For some phrases, such as "I am OK", the appropriate simple opposite phrases are hard to find or decide upon. You need to test negative phrases using an opposite and yet without using negative words in the phrase, such as "not" or "don't". Look for phrases like strong/weak, happy/sad, and healthy/sick. The statement "*not* OK" isn't really the opposite of OK, it's more like the absence of OK-ness you might say, rather than the opposite of OK. It's important to keep both the positive and negative testing statements positively framed, and clearly reflective of both the positive and negative states of the same issue. That way you can test them both equally. Occasionally I've used a single positive or negative word or phrase by itself, such as "I am OK", just to check it out, and did so in both tenses. That is, using all four phrases reflecting the two tenses and two time frames: "I am…", "I am completely…", "I will be…", and "I will be completely…".

The dictionary opposite of "okay" is "unacceptable" or "unsatisfactory" - so you can test those words, or make up your own more suitable phrase which must be what-for-you is the opposite of OK.

Occasionally, to assist myself in locating issues that I might be unaware of, I tested all sorts of negative words and phrases to see how they tested. If anything tested strongly in the negative, such as "I am ugly" for example, before correcting it I would first decide on what was the most appropriate opposite positive phrase, such as: "I am beautiful", and then test and correct the positive phrase before proceeding to re-test and correct the negative phrase - testing in both tenses, for a total of four phrases for each new test.

I kept checking to see if I was strong or weak when saying (and tuning my **TF** to) various words or phrases that had the potential to be emotionally loaded, and then I proceeded to do whatever corrections were necessary, following the same basic procedures as outlined above for **correcting basic reversals**.

Explorative self-testing was one of the main reasons I had sought to develop a 100% reliable method of self-testing, so I was thrilled to be able to finally get to work on tidying up the far corners of my inner rooms – a few of which had some pretty old used and abused junk lying around in there. And, oh the dust! ☺

Over many days, I worked steadily on testing and correcting my **PRs** and writing down what I was testing, and noticing which issues were calling for more than reversal correction. Issues requiring further in-depth treatment, with either TFT Algorithms or TFT Diagnosis. It's fairly easy to tell which things need further treatment, and as difficult as some issues can be, the good news is that you can actually self-treat them and eliminate their ill-effects.

HOW TO KNOW IF A PROBLEM REQUIRES TFT TREATMENT:

Using a **1-10 feel-bad scale**, with 10 reflecting the highest degree of distress, and 1 reflecting the lowest degree of distress, it is possible to measure how badly you feel when thinking of a particular problem. This 1 to 10 measurement reflects a subjective level (or unit) of distress you feel while thinking of that problem. And that **s**ubjective **u**nit of **d**istress you feel is called your **SUD** level, for short. So, if you have an issue, any issue, that when you think of it you feel a **s**ubjective **u**nit of **d**istress which you can measure on a scale of 1 to 10, then that measurable distress is called your **SUD** level.

When measuring your **SUD** level, it's important to use a reality-based scale such that 10 means the worst possible, flat out, incapacitating sort of distress, and 1 means the lowest possible, or no perceivable distress. If you recall our friend Al at the beginning of this manual, he reported a SUD of 10 when thinking of his problem, which was an extreme fear of heights. The minute he tuned his **TF** to the problem he actually broke out in sweat, turned a deathly pallor, and felt queasy and weak. His reaction was for him a full-on 10. After treatment, it was equally clear that his SUD had fallen to a 1, because he was calm and relaxed, his color was pink and healthy, and most importantly, he reported that his SUD had gone down to a 1. He was free of distress while thinking of the same problem that only a few moments before had caused his SUD to rise up uncontrollably to a frightening and near-incapacitating 10.

So, let's say you have a fear of something such that when you think about it in present time, you can feel your SUD level begin to rise. That's a pretty good indication that TFT treatment is needed, and if done correctly, would likely be of great benefit. Any SUD level can be treated with TFT, and **the general goal of TFT treatment** is to reduce that **SUD** level to a 2 or lower, on a scale of 1 to 10. It would be smart and beneficial to treat any problem that has an accompanying SUD of 2 or higher. If you know beforehand that a certain problem likely has a high SUD level, you needn't tune to it for long – just enough to begin applying the most appropriate algorithm for reducing it.

If you are already a TFT practitioner then you know how to treat your own fears, for example, with a TFT algorithm. If, however, you are not a TFT practitioner and you would like to be able to self-treat your own fear or anxiety, then you would proceed to use a TFT Algorithm specifically designed to treat fear, phobia, and anxiety at various levels of intensity from 1 to 10. In this case, to treat a fear you would use the same Algorithm that I used on Al at the beginning of this manual. By attending a weekend TFT Algorithm class, you can learn them all.

HOW TO SELF-TREAT WITH THE TFT ANXIETY ALGORITHM:

It's very simple really. My four and six year old clients and most of my grandchildren know how to self treat with this algorithm. First, you tune your Thought Field to the problem, and assess your SUD level on a scale of 1 to 10. Then you begin applying the TFT Algorithm of your choice directly to the appropriate spots on your body. In this case, the Algorithm for fear/anxiety/phobia is to tap **under your eye, under your arm, and on your collarbone point, consecutively.** Like this:

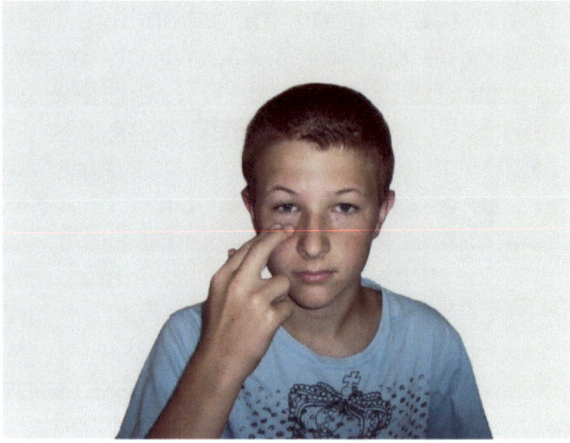

e

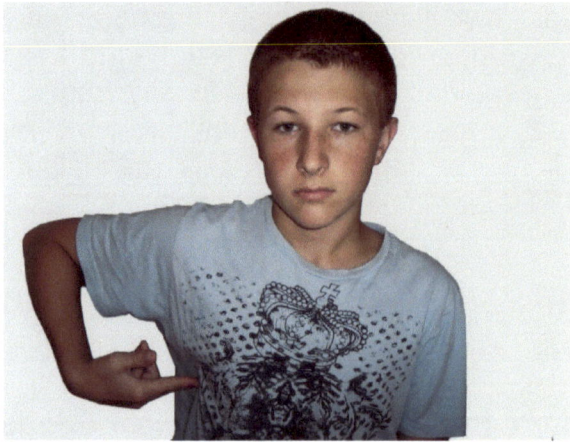

a

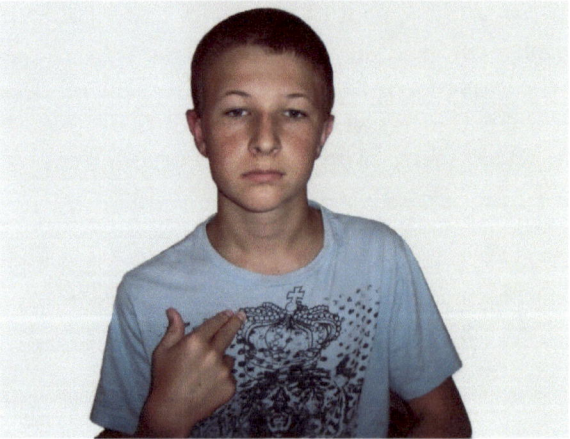

c

Then, you follow that sequence of spots (**e,a,c**) with a series of moves called the **9 Gamut**, which includes **9 specific movements** done while tapping the Gamut spot on the back of one of your hands. And after that, you're going to repeat the initial sequence of spots (**e,a,c**) again – just as we did with AI.

Here's the **Gamut spot**. It's located on the back of the hand, between the 4th and 5th fingers, just behind the knuckles and between the tendons, where there's a natural dip.

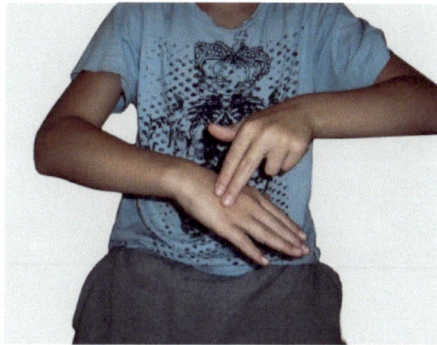

HOW TO DO THE 9 GAMUT SERIES OF MOVES: while *continuously* tapping the Gamut spot on the back of one of your hands (either hand), do these 9 specific movements at the same time: (It's easier than patting your head and rubbing your tummy at the same time! ☺)

Start tapping and…

1) close your eyes
2) open your eyes
3) look downward toward one elbow
4) look downward toward the other elbow
5) whirl your eyes in a big circle in one direction (full frame of your eye socket)
6) whirl your eyes in a big circle in the opposite direction
7) hum five notes out loud, musically (any tune will do)
8) count to five out loud, mathematically
9) hum five notes out loud, musically

Now, repeat the same sequence that you did at the beginning of the Algorithm, which is to tap **under eye, under arm, and collarbone point.**

OK. That's one round of the anxiety algorithm. Algorithms, in TFT at least, are kind of like a sandwich, with the repeated treatment points being like 2 slices of bread, and the 9 Gamut series of moves being like the filling.

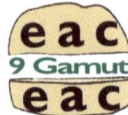

So, now that you've done one round of the standard anxiety algorithm, you need to re-assess your **SUD** to see how far it went down, because this measurement tells you how specifically to proceed with the treatment.

Following and eliminating the SUD:

1) If your SUD went down 2 or more points, repeat the entire algorithm, and re-assess again. Then, if it moves down 2 or more points again, **repeat and reassess until the SUD is down to a 2 or less.**

2) If it did not move at all, or moved only 1 point, then tap the side of your hand, and repeat the entire Algorithm. If it then moves 2 or more points, you go back to #1 (above) and follow the instructions again.

If, however, it still doesn't move, or moves only 1 point (rather than 2 or more), you will need to do an exercise called the **Collarbone Breathing** exercise, which will assist in speeding up the process of reducing your SUD. The Collarbone Breathing exercise is explained on page 53 directly after the **Floor to Ceiling Eye Roll** exercise.

Once you do the **Collarbone Breathing** exercise, you then resume the same algorithm you were using, by repeating #1 above. Repeat the same algorithm as many times as is necessary to take your **SUD** level down to a 2 or below. Be persistent and tenacious about bringing the SUD down. Since you're dealing with your own **TF**, you can create all the time you need to self-treat, and you can stay with it until you get the result you want - refusing to accept anything less than complete removal of the problem. Therefore, as needed, keep repeating the process (#1 and #2 above) until your SUD level is down to a 2 or lower. Two points lower per each application of an algorithm would require a minimum of four complete rounds of the algorithm to get to a SUD of 2. Often however, the SUD will jump much faster and further, and you may only need to do the algorithm once or twice to eliminate the problem entirely.

3) Once your SUD level is down to a 2 or below, you then finish or close the treatment by doing the **Floor-to-ceiling Eye Roll** exercise as instructed below.

FLOOR TO CEILING EYE-ROLL EXERCISE:

Casually called **"the Eye-roll"** or **"ER"** amongst **TFT'ers**, this exercise is simple, easy, and a great thing to do whenever first feeling anxious about anything while your **SUD** is still low. In any Thought Field, before your SUD rises past a 2, doing the Eye-roll will usually bring it down and also keep it from rising higher, if repeated as needed. As well, **the Eye-roll is used to complete all TFT treatments.** As soon as the SUD of any specific problem has been brought down to a 2 or lower, the treatment is followed by the **Eye-roll**.

So, whether at the end of an algorithm, or before requiring an algorithm, as soon as a **SUD** level is at a 2, whether it's a SUD on the way up or on the way down, doing the Eye-roll will help reduce that SUD level before it has a chance to rise up. However, if it does rise, then it's a call for treatment using a TFT Algorithm or TFT Diagnosis.

The Eye-roll is easy to do. You can be standing or sitting. You can even do it in public (like at the airport) and no one will notice…they'll think you're looking at something on the ceiling or the floor.

THE EYE-ROLL: sit in a normal seated position with your head still and facing forward. Now start tapping the Gamut spot continuously (either hand will do as you're going to tap both hands) while keeping your head still and facing forward. Then roll your eyes straight down as far as they will go, and slowly begin to raise them upward toward the ceiling over your head, while still tapping the Gamut spot, and while keeping your head steady and only moving your eyes.

Once you have rolled your eyes all the way up and back into your head so to speak, hold them there for a second and then relax, allowing your eyes to return to their normal position.

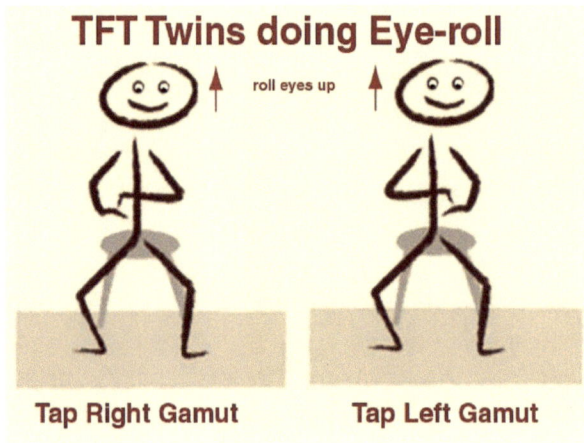

TFT Twins doing Eye-roll

roll eyes up

Tap Right Gamut   **Tap Left Gamut**

Then switch hands and start tapping the Gamut spot on your other hand, and repeat the exact same Eye-roll exercise while tapping the new hand. In other words, you do the exercise twice - once on each hand.

That's the end of the **Eye-roll** exercise.

THE COLLARBONE BREATHING EXERCISE: You need to do this exercise whenever your SUD level, during self-treatment, decreases slowly, moving down by only one point rather than two or more.

At first glance, this exercise seems a bit more complex to learn than the others, however, once you do it a couple of times, it goes quickly and smoothly offering noticeable and on-going benefits. With a continuous tap, I can do this exercise with successful results, in just over 30 seconds – though it takes 3-5 minutes when you're first learning how to do it.

Here's a sneak preview prior to following the instructions below: you're going to be doing a specific breathing pattern while at the same time touching the Collarbone point on one side of your body and tapping the back of that hand with your other hand. Then, you're going to bend the fingers of your touching hand, and repeat the same tapping and breathing pattern while those fingers are bent. Then, you're going to do the exact same thing while touching the other Collarbone point. And then (as if that were not enough ☺), you're going to switch hands and repeat everything all over again on both sides of your body.

HOW TO DO COLLARBONE BREATHING:

Part A

1) Place the first 2 fingers of one hand on one of your collarbone points (either **cb** point will do). It looks like you're pointing at your chest, so let's call this your 'pointer' hand.

You'll be using both hands and both **cb** points during this exercise, so it doesn't matter which side you start with, just touch your one of your collarbone points with the first 2 fingers of one of your hands.

2) Then, with the first 2 fingers of your other hand, which we'll call your 'tapping' hand, you begin *continuously tapping* the Gamut spot on the back of your 'pointing' hand. Like this:

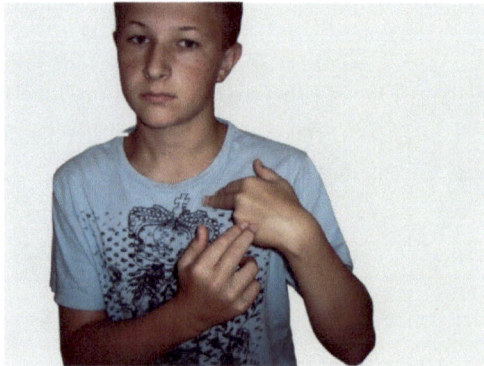

3) Now, while still ***continuously tapping*** the Gamut spot (a continuous tap means you needn't count - simply tap, breathe, and hold your breath for about 5 taps or more, for each hand position) and **follow this meditative-like breathing pattern at the same time as you're tapping (it's calming and pleasant)**:

First, **breathe normally** for 5 taps
Then, **breathe all the way in** and **hold your breath** for 5 taps
Then, **breathe halfway out**, and **hold your breath** for 5 taps.
Then, **breathe all the way out**, and **hold your breath** for 5 taps.
Then, **breathe half way in,** and **hold your breath** for 5 taps.
That's it.

Now, you're going to make a slight adjustment of your 'pointing' hand by bending the 2 pointed fingers so that your knuckles are now resting (or kneeling) on that same collarbone point, rather than pointed fingers on the point. Then you repeat the same tapping and breathing moves as above (steps 2 & 3) with bent knuckles, while tapping the Gamut spot on the back of your same 'pointing' hand. Like this:

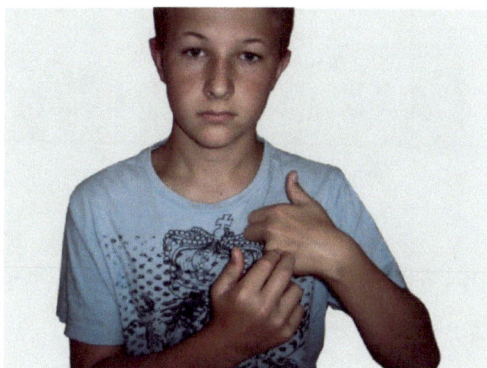

Now that you've done the breathing and tapping with straight and bent fingers on one side of your chest, you're going to do the very same thing on the other side, so that you'll have done it on both sides, which means on both **cb** points. Like this:

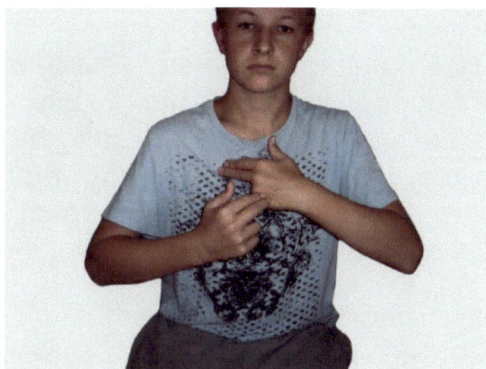

Simply lift up both hands and move them to the other side, touching the other **cb** point with the same two fingers of the same 'pointing' hand, doing the tapping and breathing exactly as above, and then repeating the tapping and breathing with bent knuckles also. Like this:

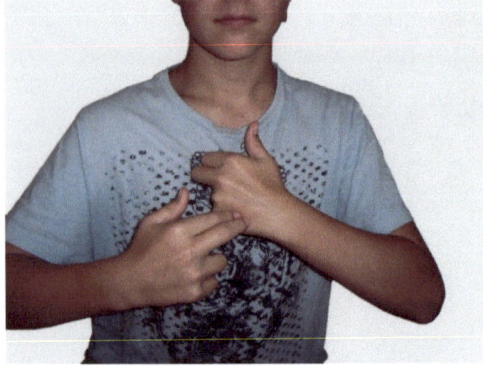

OK. Now you've tapped and breathed with pointed and bent fingers on both cb points, which means you've completed part A of the **CB** exercise, and are ready for part B.

Part B

1) Repeat Part A doing everything exactly the same except starting with the opposite 'pointing' hand from which you started in Part A.

Repeat steps 1,2,3,& 4, doing everything the same, using your new 'pointing' hand as the leader.

In short, start with the first two fingers of your new 'pointing' hand touching one of your collarbone points (it doesn't matter which one because you're going to use both), and begin tapping the Gamut spot on the back of your new **'pointing'** hand with 2 fingers of your new **'tapping'** hand. Then, **repeat instruction 3 & 4** above, just as you did before when starting with your first 'pointing' hand.

Now that you've completed the Collarbone Breathing exercise, if you were doing the **CB** exercise because you were in the middle of an anxiety (or other) self-treatment that was moving slowly, you would now return and complete that same self-treatment. For the standard TFT anxiety treatment turn to **page 46**.

Or, if you were doing **CB** on its own because of a perceived need such as clumsiness, feeling spaced out, feeling toxic, or having dyslexic or reading difficulties, then you would simply do **CB** and return to the rest of your day.

Whenever a TFT self-treatment is going slower than expected, do the **CB** exercise and then continue on with your self-treatment. You will find that doing the **CB** exercise creates a further jump in the reduction of the **SUD** level, making the treatment progress faster.

As well, do the **CB** exercise whenever you feel a perceived need to do it. That is, whenever you're feeling clumsy, knocking your elbows on door frames, feeling spaced out, disconnected, have poor concentration, or feeling toxic. First correct your **PRs**, and then do the **CB** exercise. CB is thought to assist with neurological imbalance.

XXII

Speaking of things moving slowly reminds me of our fellow in the monastery. By now he had been studying diligently for months and months, and every few weeks the old Master would come into his room and ask him the same question. And each time he would tell the Master that he still did not know everything there was to know. And each time the Master would raise his staff and begin beating the man about the head and shoulders, and then leave.

Eventually one day, while he was studying ever diligently, the old master came into his room, and asked him again: "Have you learned everything there is to know?"

"No." said the man, "I have not."

At which point the master raised his staff high into the air, but this time the man thrust out his arm and caught the staff in the crux of his open hand. At which point the Master paused...and then burst out with a mighty laugh.

"Why are you laughing?" said the man, "I have failed. I will never know everything there is to know!"

"Yes," said the master. "That is true. I'm laughing for joy, because today you have learned two things. One, you will never know everything there is to know. And two, how to stop the pain."

SELF-CORRECTION WITHOUT SELF-TESTING:

You can and should self-test and self-treat for PR whenever you notice its effects, whenever you suspect it, are feeling badly, or your thoughts are reflexively negative. And you can also correct for PR without testing it every time, simply by tapping the side of your hand a few times a day (15-20 taps each time) every day, for the great benefit it offers, regardless of a perceived need to do it.

And you can do the same with **CB** breathing by doing it twice a day, every day, for the great benefit it offers, regardless of a perceived need to do it.

Doing these two TFT exercises a few times a day, every day, has the potential to alter your life for the better in countless seen and unseen ways. You will be able to appreciate the change as soon as you start doing them every day. You can also test and correct specific reversals as they show up in your thinking, and do whatever further self-treatment with **TFT Algorithms** that suits your needs at any time. As well, you can use the NRG Method with any other healing modalities, whenever and wherever muscle-testing is used.

THE BENEFITS OF ACCURATE SELF-MUSCLE-TESTING:

….are, I think it's safe to say, *HUGE!!!*

Imagine, for example, that you have just stepped off an airplane in which the person sitting beside you was wearing a chemical-based perfume or deodorant that made you feel poorly. Perhaps your good energy dropped and your mood went down, or you got a pain behind your eyes, or you felt a migraine threatening.

Clearly, one or more ingredients in the scent you were exposed to affected you adversely, negatively. In fact, for you, that scent was a toxin, and your reaction to it is your immediate feed-back experience of your body cells and systems being affected by that toxin.

So, you get off the plane feeling lousy, pale, and miffed at the 'perpetrator'. You need to be in good form for a business meeting in an hour, or perhaps you have a dinner date with a new romantic partner, or a family reunion, or (yikes!) a stage performance. Grrrr, what're ya gonna do…?

The standard available options are to take pain-killers, anti-inflammatory drugs, cancel your engagements, find a TFT VT practitioner in a hurry, or…*what if* you knew how to use the NRG self-muscle-testing method that allows you to use a small gym weight to self-test, and some basic TFT to self-treat, and in that way you can set yourself straight in minutes.

So, you find a place to sit or stand, and begin testing and treating yourself with TFT to eliminate the ill effects of the toxin you were exposed to, or the food you ate, etc.

You don't have a gym weight with you, so you use your water bottle as a weight, or your briefcase – it doesn't matter, as long as it's a good weight for you to get a solid test. Having learned to self-muscle-test accurately means you already know exactly what size weight is best for you, and how to use it to get an accurate test, and so finding the right size water bottle or rock is easy enough.

Within minutes, you've tested and corrected yourself for the standard TFT 'reversals', and you've treated yourself with TFT's brilliant 7 Second Toxin Treatment for 'that scent', and you've brought your reaction down from a feel bad 7 to a feel good 0-2. Phew! You're feeling good again, and you look better too - fresh, maybe even glowing.

You think: "Thank God for TFT and for Self-Muscle-Testing!" and you go on your way. No ill-effects of pain-killing drugs, no migraine, no exhaustion, no down time.

Had you not known how to accurately self-muscle-test, or how to use TFT to correct your 'reversals' or treat your toxin-reactive state, this story and your day would have likely been a lot different, and far more stressful – even disastrous.

For those who already know TFT, or who are TFT therapists, there are many ways in which knowing how to self-muscle-test accurately provides you with an added remarkable tool. For example, you can use it not only to test and correct yourself, but also to test and correct others, surrogate-ly. That is, you can test a baby or animal or immobile person, by using a weight to test yourself as a surrogate for them, while you're either touching their body, or listening to their voice.

You can use self-muscle-testing to correct not only your own and others' reversals, you can also use it to select the best TFT algorithms, or select single points, or a combination of points to more completely resolve a problem.

You can use self-muscle-testing to check your supplements, foods, drinks and products BEFORE you ingest or smell them, or alas, afterwards, to correct a negative reaction.

You can treat yourself for all sorts of negative emotional states and feelings, as well as past traumatic events that you might otherwise never get around to actually resolving. Those various issues that may not be quite bad enough to get you to a therapist, or quite good enough to be permitted to remain in a healthy thought field. In fact, you can use self-muscle-testing and TFT to clean up your entire thought field if you like, creating a clean and well-lit place to really 'be'.

THE TIME HAS COME

The combination of self-muscle-testing with **The NRG Method** and applying TFT protocols to self-treat, gives you the tools you need to make huge changes in all areas of your life - your thought field, your mind, your emotions, your spiritual self, and your physical self too - positively affecting the quality of your entire life now and into the future. There are TFT algorithms for fear, pain, anger, trauma, grief, obsession, love pain, guilt, shame, depression, jet lag, anxiety, rage, physical pain, addiction, turbulence, panic, embarrassment, and more. And there are lots of TFT practitioners available to further assist you if needed, including myself: www.NRGHolistic.com

Now that you've learned **the NRG Method** of self-muscle-testing, the power to heal yourself is in your hands.

Why, a few months from now, and on into time, your life can be pleasantly and seamlessly altered, turned around, refurbished, back on track, and heightened beyond measure – feeling more like your own self, once again.

You can do it! ☺

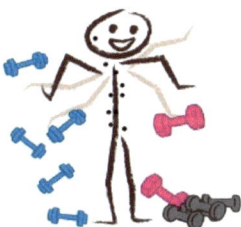

…the beginning

TESTIMONIALS

I received these testimonials after treating clients, by phone, with my Whole Body Protocols, including unique natural supplements, constitutional Homeopathy, TFT Voice Technology, and in some cases with distance healing techniques as well.

From a Canadian author: (**Trigeminal Nerve Shingles**)

The pain from acute shingles prompted me to seek help from Norma Gairdner, H.D. Within 20 minutes of TFT by telephone, the severe pain disappeared, never to return. The word miracle came to mind! The combination of Norma's intensive training, her insights, modern technology, and ancient wisdom provides consistent and lasting relief from myriad illnesses and conditions. (R.S., Toronto)

From an artist and writer: (**Complex Trauma**)

I am seventy two years old and it seems I spent my entire lifetime in therapy. However, in only two days of Thought Field Therapy with Norma Gairdner my life was transformed. All of the issues that I had thrashed over with conventional therapists evaporated within a couple of sessions with Norma. Now, I do the simple treatments that she introduced me to and voila, there is a space of clarity and peace before me that is hard to describe - a total absence of everything stressful, a void that feels so precious it's difficult to describe. I thank you, the creators of TFT, for this incredible advent into emotional healing and I celebrate Norma's magnificence in applying it. (P.W., Colorado)

From a singer, writer, performer: (**Complex Trauma & love pain**)

Norma helped me through a time of shattering on every level of my life. Whenever panic and negativity overwhelmed me, she was there with treatments that calmed the inner storms and encouraged healing. I don't know how I would have made it through my dark night of the soul without her. Thank you, Norma. (B.M., Montana)

<u>From a Mental Health & International Relief Worker</u>: (**Taught him the NRG Method of self-muscle-testing**)

Clearly, Dr. Norma Gairdner has added a new dimension to the muscle testing technique so necessary for determining the presence of psychological reversal (PR) and the impact of toxins. Her personal technique of self-muscle-testing, along with Callahan TFT protocols, makes self-treatment easy and effective, and now I don't have to depend on anyone else to muscle-test me. Thank you, Dr.Gairdner for your innovative way of helping us help ourselves. (H.A.,Washington)

<u>From a world-renowned Canadian Orthopaedic surgeon</u>: (**Parkinson's Disease**)

I am a physician educated in Western medicine. In recent years however, I have become familiar with Homeopathy and Thought Field Therapy through the care of Norma Gairdner. I have a progressive neuromuscular condition, Parkinson's Disease, for which there are few effective therapies - often only symptomatic or palliative relief. I do believe that through the treatments of Norma Gairdner, I now have a steadier gate, less tremor, and a deeper sleep each night. I am improved, without drugs, and we only just started. (Written five years prior to a fatal fall - Dr. Robert Salter, Toronto.)

<u>From a Designer</u>: (**Chronic Insomnia**)

I want to thank you for your tremendous help in assisting me in getting my sleeping pattern back on track, as it was taking a toll on my life. The medical solution was drugs which I used initially out of desperation and ignorance. Then I came to Norma to find a homeopathic solution to my problem. Within a few weeks, and off the medication, my length of sleeping gradually increased to a point where I actually slept an entire night, for the first time in several years - what a celebration. Norma guided me through Homeopathic and Thought Field Therapy to regain control over my sleep patterns. And now, almost a year later I can honestly say that I have not had a recurrence and sleep peacefully every night. Thank you Norma !!!!!!!!!! (P.S., Toronto)

From a Decorator: (**Fear of flying**)

Just weeks before an important business trip, I was so consumed with the fear of flying that I almost wanted to quit my job. My anxiety levels had reached a fever pitch, and I was living an acute and over-sensitized life, over-reacting to even small things. I was doing everything I could to keep control of the things in my life, but was always under fear of losing it, all spurred on by a sudden phobia of flying that I had never really had before. I finally sought the help of Norma Gairdner, who I worked with for 2 weeks prior to my flight. As a result of Norma's therapy, I was able to breathe again, feel under control, and sleep restfully again. Connectedness to others came back, and most of all, balance. With her program, I was able to get to the airport, meet colleagues in the lounge, have relaxing conversation, and board the plane to take my seat. Once seated, I read a magazine in total calmness and with a sense of security. I did not experience the anticipated panic attack at all, and this was at once a complete wonderment and a welcome development. Norma changed so much for me for the better. Thank you! (C.C, Toronto)

From a photographer and homebuilder: (**Chronic irregular heartbeat**)

For years my heart has been of concern to me. Having been diagnosed with a prolapsed mitral valve years ago, to the doctors reversing that diagnosis and finally determining I had lone atrial fib and extra beats. The doctors said to either "get used to my irregular beats" which were keeping me awake and waking me up constantly throughout the night, or to "take beta blockers". I asked Norma to help me, and upon giving me a homeopathic remedy and 20 minutes of TFT. I have been so pleased, and for the past year without hardly any symptoms. I felt so terrible on beta blockers and now, thanks to Norma, I feel great. (C.G., Ontario)

<u>From a mother</u>: (4 yr old boy with whole-body itching bleeding **Eczema**.)

From my point of view, this treatment has given me back my son, who is nearly completely better at this writing. We barely had any relationship outside of the confrontations surrounding his intense desire to scratch and my trying to prevent him from scratching. Now we interact on many other levels. He seems much more peaceful, both mentally and physically. I hear about his day at school, we make up stories together, draw pictures together, and I am now able to cuddle with him more, especially at bedtime as he can stay still longer. During the times when the eczema was the worst, he pulled away from me and our energies reminded me of two magnets with opposite polarities repelling each other. He would thrash about so that I was risking injury to be near him. Tonight he told me that his favourite thing now is snuggling. What a precious gift to be able to hold my son again. Words cannot express my gratitude, Norma. Thank you. (L.F., Ontario)

<u>Re my mentor</u>: Roger J. Callahan, PhD - Founder, Thought Field Therapy.

My ageing husband suffered from **chronic and sometimes acute bronchitis**. After years of recurring prescriptions for antibiotics, and numerous homeopathic protocols, Norma got it under control and he never had to take another round of antibiotics. None of the other homeopaths we went to achieved the same immediate response or sustained level of results.

But even more importantly, her expertise greatly improved his overall quality of life. She was able to ease the challenges of being in one's late 80's; relieving aches and pains, and balance and mobility issues, and digestive difficulties, whenever she was called upon, and all without the risky side-effects of medications. Norma is a wizard with homeopathy, TFT, and nutritional support. We were both very grateful for her care, and I still consult her for all my general health needs. I never hesitate to heartily recommend her to our clients. (Joanne Callahan, President, Callahan Techniques.)

<u>From a mother</u>: (twin boys diagnosed with **Autism** at 18 months)

Our twin sons were placed on the Autism Disorder Spectrum when they were 18 months old. They showed signs of major delay with no walking or talking (extremely vocal, but had no language), and they lacked common communication skills like pointing and clapping. After very slow and gradual progression they began walking on their own at 20 mos., but by 26 mos. they still had no language, even though they were in private speech therapy.

Norma Gairdner, H.D., began treating my sons when they were 26 mos. She began with Thought Field Therapy (TFT), treating them for various traumas and identifying toxins and sensitivities to things the boys were regularly consuming, or being exposed to, such as scented laundry products and air fresheners. After doing TFT with them, the boys' general behavior and temperament seemed to change within that hour. With a schedule of homeopathic remedies, elimination of various foods and chemicals, and lots of TFT (most often by phone), their language became recognizable and a gush of new words began to come from them daily.

Norma's treatments have not only opened up the huge dam that was blocking the boys' development, but her unyielding dedication and relentless research into supportive and corrective supplements, cutting edge literature and progressive websites, to aid in further discovering a curative treatment has been irrevocably and ultimately appreciated.

There are no true words to express our debt of gratitude to her as we had ultimately felt that our twins' "sentence" was for life, and looking around at the limited resources that western medicine recognizes, we began to have no hope for recovery. Now, we see the light at the end of the tunnel, and it's all because of Norma's guiding hand, knowledge and determination. Today, the boys are 3.5 years old. They are walking, and talking (*all* the time), and both boys are extremely social and loving to everyone around them. It is expected by their pediatrician that they will be removed from the Autism Disorder Spectrum in July 2010, at their next Neurological Pediatrician appointment.

With love and admiration. (A.M., Ontario. March 2010)

N.B. The boys were removed from the Autism Spectrum by their M.D., in July 2010. They entered kindergarten in the fall. Spring 2011, mother reports: **"They're thriving!"**

From the mother of my interpreter when teaching advanced personal awareness seminars, in Moscow: I treated her mother, whom I had never met, using distance healing techniques, followed by one dose of a constitutional homeopathic remedy: (**Chronic disease state**)

My name is A. B. I am 70 years old. I live in the South of Russia. For the last 30-35 years I am suffering from a severe form of drug allergy. My case is complicated with chronic pyelonephritis, chronic pancreatitis, chronic gastritis, varicose veins, cerebral stroke and other deceases, such as basal cell carcinoma on my right eyelid. In December 2005 I was very sick. I felt enormous weakness, apathy, high fever, and sadness. Besides, I had a high blood pressure (240/100), and a bad pyelonephritis attack. I cannot explain how badly I felt. Norma (she is friend with my daughter) was so kind to agree to take my case and to treat me with TFT in a distance from Canada to Russia. As a result of Norma's treatment I felt 30-35% better during the first session, and my fever came right down. She worked on me everyday until I was 90% better, and my blood pressure came to a normal 130/80. It has not been normal for many, many years. As well, I became buoyant, and even began to react on jokes. Up until now - today, one year later - I am still feeling myself well and buoyant. I do a lot of things in the house and in my garden that I have not been able to do for many years. Even if I get tired physically, I am still buoyant and happy to be alive. I am deeply impressed by the method Norma used for treating me - especially all the way from Canada to Russia. It is a miracle how it worked! (A.B., North Ossetia.)

From an author and Medical Science writer: (**Abdominal Mass in 87 year old**)

I attribute the disappearance of a large palpable mass in my abdomen to the powerful healing intervention of Norma Gairdner, H.D. The mass, two inches in diameter, was witnessed by family, and by family physician, and clearly visible in ultrasound.
Norma is an extraordinary healer, skilled in many modes of healing including Homeopathy and Thought Field Therapy (TFT). (S.R., Ontario)

From a father: (10 year old son, **Tourette Syndrome**)

We started working with Norma in January 2012, a few months after confirmation of our son's diagnosis of Tourette Syndrome. At the time, our son J's physical tics and involuntary vocalizations were increasing in intensity, and becoming almost seizure-like, with eyes rolling back into his head. However, with Norma's guidance to alter his diet, probiotic treatment, elimination of toxins and chemicals from our home, constitutional homeopathy and on-going TFT treatment, he rapidly made substantial and remarkable improvements that have endured in the long term. At this time, and for 4 to 5 months now, J has been consistently between 85-100% better in all areas of measurement.
We are very grateful for Norma's holistic approach to our son's treatment, and her deep understanding of his healing needs as a patient. (M.N., Ontario)

From a mother: (9 year old daughter, **severe Autism**)

My daughter M was diagnosed with autism at the age of 3. This was very devastating to our whole family and especially to me as a parent. We had tried many, many treatments in the last 6 years and we sought Norma's help originally for cease therapy. We only have just started her treatments but we have seen improvements in many areas already. We have seen 70-80% improvement in her joint attention, and significant improvement in her sleeping habits, M used to sleep no more that 4-5 hours at night with a lot of disruptive behavior. Norma brought to our attention that the detergents and perfumes we were using were a problem. After 1 week of a scent-free home we have seen an 95% improvement in her sleep and night time behaviors. We have also seen gains in her nutrition – after weighing 50 pounds for ages and ages, she has suddenly gained 8 pounds already! We have seen a great improvement in her gait and balance. Although we still have far to go we are optimistic for the first time in a long time. Thank you Norma (M.F., Ontario)

<u>From a homemaker</u>: (**Complex Trauma**, **PTSD**.)

I have been attempting to fix myself since I was in my early twenties. I have been from pillar to post...therapists, shrinks, every self-help book and program both free and highly expensive. During those long painful years I learned some things and this is one of the things I'd very much like to pass to you, Norma: of all the books, pills, shrinks, meditating, humming, praying, etc., that I have done, YOU stand out as the most helpful, effective, and fast fast fast relief from painful memories and self-destructive tendencies. Your healing practices, and (dare I say it) psychic abilities, and further a spirituality that is non-denominational....and also, you are not afraid to get in there and call a spade a spade. I needed that. I know when I call you that within minutes I will feel better. No one has ever been able to do this. Thank you thank you thank you. (D.B.,Toronto)

<u>From a mother</u>: (19 year old son, Autsm) Treated son for **ASD** & mother for **Chronic Fatigue, IBS, and PTSD**.)

I had raised my autistic son for 18 years, with the help of many good and not so good therapies, therapists, teachers, and care givers. When I found Norma, my son was still pacing and hand-clenching, fearful, and not wanting to be touched. My biggest wish was that he graduate from the high school program he was in, and somehow go on to function more independently at whatever he might do after high school. As it turned out, I got my wish and more so! The pacing and hand clenching are gone, he has graduated from high school, he got a driver's license, and is living on his own at college studying music! A well-earned miracle!!!
Thankfully, Norma treated me as well: after 20 years of stomach problems and many efforts to find the most effective treatments, I finally have lasting relief from pain, and the constraints of living with an unpredictable illness. All gone!!! No longer worry about sudden painful bouts followed by crushing fatigue, and I can regularly enjoy foods I thought I would never be able to touch again.
Clearly, the results have been life changing for both of us!!! (A.G., Toronto)

<u>From a Visionary, Artist, Film maker, & Inventor</u>: **(Marginal Zone Lymphoma)**

In 2011, I was diagnosed with a low grade form of Lymphoma. My energy was debilitatingly low, and just getting dressed required several breaks. My older sister had died of Lymphoma a few years before, and my oldest son had years ago luckily survived Hodgkin's Lymphoma, however, it looked and definitely felt like I was at the beginning of my way out. The Oncology ward at our local hospital, monitored my state on a regular basis. In the year before I came under Norma's care little had changed. Thanks to the guidance of holistic healer Norma Gairdner, H.D., who uses Homeopathy, TFT voice technology, and whole body nutritional protocols, my way back to health also included dietary changes, powerful probiotics, and removal of offending causes. Fortunately, I never had to do chemo or radiation. A year later, as I turned 75, the best gift was the Oncologist report that my blood count was back to normal and there were "no signs of the lymphoma"! I think I already knew that because my energy had come back - not like it was at 18 - but better than it's been in a long time. Thanks Norma, I have a renewed lease and maybe some time to finish all these projects! (Bill Lishman, Ontario)

<u>From a Psychologist</u>: (Treated her husband who was **gravely ill** from too long awaiting transplant.)

Norma is a true healer. She uses a combination of effective, cutting-edge methods, along with a keen sense of intuition. I truly believe that my husband is alive today because of her work with him at a distance. Her caring comes through in all that she does. (J.E., Colorado)

Norma Ruth Gairdner, M.A., H.D., TFT-Adv

As a 21st century medicine woman, health and wellbeing coach, personal awareness trainer, mother, grandmother, and teacher, Norma employs a variety of unique healing modalities to assist and comfort, with intent toward healthful change and renewed authenticity and freedom. Many of her clients experience robust transformation to spirited models of health and wellbeing, echoing the phrase: "I feel like myself again."

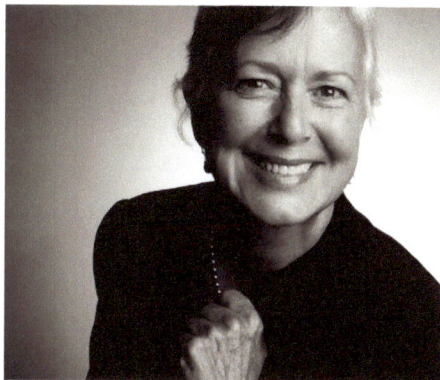

Following an M.A. in English and years of postgraduate interdisciplinary study, Norma traveled far to study with original founders and top teachers of many new and ancient healing modalities including Massage Therapy, Polarity Therapy, T'ai Chi Chuan, Lomi Deep Tissue, Tellington Touch, Rebirthing, Whole Brain Functioning, Shamanism, Soul Retrieval, New Decision Therapy, Reconnective Healing, Quantum Touch, Thought Field Therapy (TFT-Adv), CEASE Therapy (for ASDs), and of course, Homeopathic Medicine.

After graduating with honors from the International Academy of Homeopathy and the Homeopathic College of Canada, she became Clinic Supervisor of the Teaching Clinic of the HCC, teaching first year Homeopathic Medicine and the course for M.D.s and health professionals. In 1998, she was elected President of the Ontario Homeopathic Association and was responsible for the completion and submission of the application for regulation of the homeopathic profession to the Government of Ontario. Through the OHA, Norma is registered as a Doctor of Homeopathy (H.D.) #9501. She sits on the Advisory Council of the Ontario College of Homeopathic Medicine. As a past board member of the Association for Thought Field Therapy Foundation, she formed and chaired the Trauma Relief Committee, deploying ATFT members to assist with TFT trauma relief techniques in various global disasters, and now serves on the General Advisory Council of the ATFT (Association of Thought Field Therapy).

During the years of raising a family she studied complementary healing modalities, and worked as an advanced level personal awareness trainer. In the USA, she designed and taught advanced trainings for Impact Seminars, Koyen & Associates, and Emerge Seminars. In Japan, she designed and taught advanced trainings and trained trainers and staff for Life Dynamics. In Canada, she designed and taught Life in Balance for Outcomes, Inc. And most recently taught advanced seminars for a company in Russia.

One highlight of her career is her work with singer-activist John Denver, co-founder of the Windstar Foundation. She co-designed and co-trained the Vision Quest training donated to the Windstar Foundation by ARC International, and co-designed with John Denver and Dennis Becker, the "Higher Ground" event which John delivered and performed throughout the world to forward the action toward global sustainability.

In private practice from her home near Toronto, Norma specializes in the treatment of trauma, grief, phobia, emotional distress, and stubborn symptoms in adults and children, including ASDs. Her development of the NRG Method™ of self-muscle-testing, enables her to treat successfully by phone using TFT Voice Technology, and to teach others how to self-test and self-treat with TFT. She sings in several choirs, enjoys veil painting, writing poetry, holistic health pursuits, and spending time with family and friends at home, and in Ontario's beautiful northland.

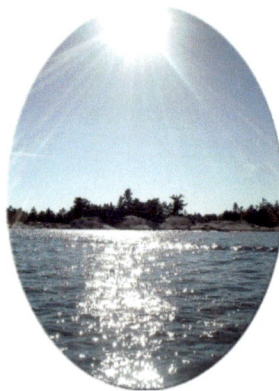